Grief Diaries

Surviving Loss by Cancer

True stories about healing and hope
after losing a loved one to cancer

LYNDA CHELDELIN FELL
with
DIANNE WEST

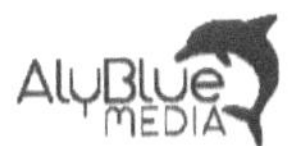

Grief Diaries
Surviving Loss by Cancer – 1st ed.
True stories about healing and hope after losing a loved one to cancer
Lynda Cheldelin Fell/Dianne West
Grief Diaries www.GriefDiaries.com

Cover Design by AlyBlue Media, LLC
Interior Design by AlyBlue Media LLC
Published by AlyBlue Media, LLC

ISBN: 978-1-944328-81-8
AlyBlue Media, LLC
Ferndale, WA 98248
www.AlyBlueMedia.com

This book is designed to provide informative narrations to readers. It is sold with the understanding that the writers, authors or publisher is not engaged to render any type of psychological, legal, or any other kind of professional advice. The content is the sole expression and opinion of the authors and writers. No warranties or guarantees are expressed or implied by the choice to include any of the content in this book. Neither the publisher nor the author or writers shall be liable for any physical, psychological, emotional, financial, or commercial damages including but not limited to special, incidental, consequential or other damages. Our views and rights are the same: You are responsible for your own choices, actions and results.

PRINTED IN THE UNITED STATES OF AMERICA

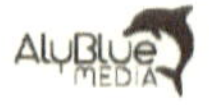

GRIEF DIARIES

Testimonials

"CRITICALLY IMPORTANT . . . I want to say to Lynda that what you are doing is so critically important." –DR. BERNICE A. KING, daughter of Dr. Martin Luther King

"INSPIRATIONAL . . . Grief Diaries is the result of heartfelt testimonials from a dedicated and loving group of people. By sharing their stories, the reader will find inspiration and a renewed sense of comfort as they move through their own journey." -CANDACE LIGHTNER, Founder of Mothers Against Drunk Driving

"DEEPLY INTIMATE . . . Grief Diaries is a deeply intimate, authentic collection of narratives that speak to the powerful, often ambiguous, and wide spectrum of emotions that arise from loss. I so appreciate the vulnerability and truth embedded in these stories." -DR. ERICA GOLDBLATT HYATT, Chair of Psychology, Bryn Athyn College

"HOPE . . . These stories reflect the authentic voices of individuals at the unexpected moment their lives were shattered and altered forever. Moments of strength in the midst of indescribable pain, resilience in the midst of rage; hope while mired in despair." —SHERIFF SADIE DARNELL, Alachua County, Florida; Chair, Florida Cold Case Advisory Commission

"BRAVE . . . The brave individuals who share their truth in this book do it for the benefit of all." CAROLYN COSTIN - Founder, Monte Nido Treatment Centers

"HOPE AND HEALING . . . You are a pioneer in this field and you are breaking the trail for others to find hope and healing." -KRISTI SMITH, Bestselling Author & International Speaker

"A FORCE . . .The writers of this project, the Grief Diaries anthology series, are a force to be reckoned with. I'm betting we will be agents of great change." -MARY LEE ROBINSON, Author and Founder of Set an Extra Plate initiative

"MOVING . . . In Grief Diaries, the stories are not only moving but often provide a rich background for any mourner to find a gem of insight that can be used in coping with loss. Re-read each story with pen in hand and you will find many that are just right for you." -DR. LOUIS LAGRAND, Author of Healing Grief, Finding Peace

"VITAL . . . Grief Diaries gives voice to the thousands who face this painful journey every day. Often alone in their time of need, these stories will play a vital role in surrounding each reader with warmth and comfort as they seek understanding and healing in the aftermath of their own loss." -JENNIFER CLARKE, R.N., Perinatal Bereavement Committee at AMITA Health Adventist Medical Center

"HEALING . . . Grief Diaries gives voice to a grief so private, most bear it alone. These diaries can heal hearts and begin to build community and acceptance to speak the unspeakable. Share this book with your sisters, mothers, grandmothers and friends who have faced grief. Pour a cup of tea together and know that you are no longer alone." -DIANNA VAGIANOS ARMENTROUT, Poetry Therapist & Author of Walking the Labyrinth of My Heart: A Journey of Pregnancy, Grief and Infant Death

"INCREDIBLE . . .Thank you so much for doing this project, it's absolutely incredible!"-JULIE MJELVE, Founder, Grieving Together

"STUNNING . . . Grief Diaries treats the reader to a rare combination of candor and fragility through the eyes of the bereaved. Delving into the deepest recesses of the heartbroken, the reader easily identifies with the diverse collection of stories and richly colored threads of profound love that create a stunning read full of comfort and hope." -DR. GLORIA HORSLEY, President, Open to Hope Foundation

"WONDERFUL . . .Grief Diaries is a wonderful computation of stories written by the best of experts, the bereaved themselves. Thank you for building awareness about a topic so near and dear to my heart." -DR. HEIDI HORSLEY, Adjunct Professor, School of Social Work, Columbia University, Author, Co-Founder of Open to Hope Organization

SURVIVING LOSS BY CANCER

Dedication

In loving memory of

John Del Vecchio
Jeff Friend
Don Horacek
Tom Hutsell
Johan Jordaan
Derek Layman
John Marchesa
Sam Cornich-Lynch
Dana Nova
Brian Pochel
Carolyn Curtiss Smith Sharp
Rob Vandervalk
Vern West

SURVIVING LOSS BY CANCER

Contents

SURVIVING LOSS BY CANCER

BY DANA BROTHERS

Introduction

Each summer, our hospice agency hosts an open bereavement educational conference. Clinicians, social workers, medical personnel, counselors, and long-term care staff attend and earn the continuing education credits needed to maintain their accreditation and licensure. Speakers teach about cutting edge research and clinical practice, and the event provides an excellent occasion for professionals to network with one another. As the Education Program Manager at Hospice of the Northwest, one of my responsibilities is to organize this event, so I am always seeking to meet experts in the grief and loss field.

While attending the annual Association for Death Education and Counseling conference, one of our medical social workers had the opportunity to meet Lynda Cheldelin Fell. She shared Lynda's contact information, which led to collaboration and a wonderful friendship.

As with many people who know Lynda, I am struck by her gentle spirit and humble presence. Even when tremendous heartache casts a shadow on her life, her face still radiates joy. I believe the principle that keeps Lynda present and connected lies in her gratitude. She understands that appreciation is essential for living the best possible life and despite the trials we may face, our resilience is the best antidote to debilitating sorrow. When she asked me to write the forward for this book, I was deeply honored. I too have been affected by cancer and believe it has directly influenced what I do in life, including my career with hospice.

My aunt Wanda was diagnosed with leiomyosarcoma, a rare soft tissue cancer, at age thirty-six. She'd been experiencing abdominal pain and nausea but with three teenagers at home, a lush garden full of plants to tend, and a husband working full time, she didn't focus on her own health. She certainly wasn't in any position to have her life end abruptly with a cancer diagnosis.

Living in a different city, we didn't visit often but, after the cancer news, that changed. I remember hushed phone conversations and my mom weeping quietly at night. I was only six years old at the time, and the word cancer scared me. All I knew was that my funny aunt, who always had fresh baked cookies, was sick.

Arriving at their home to visit a few weeks after treatment started, everything was different. My uncle was home every day, my cousins were quiet and sullen, and the kitchen smelled like antiseptic soap. An oxygen tank sat next to my aunt, and clear tubing snaked around the living room. I wanted the world to go back to the way it was, but normal was turned upside down. I later learned that after consulting on her case, a panel of eight oncologists gave my aunt a six-week prognosis; her cancer was advanced and aggressively growing.

As I read through the stories in this book, I remembered my own childhood feelings of confusion and how I yearned for normalcy. The seismic shift each family goes through when handed a cancer diagnosis was familiar. Life is divided in two: before and after diagnosis. This was true of our family, and is illustrated by each writer who bravely share their experience in this book.

Surviving Loss By Cancer sheds light on how losing a loved one to cancer changes our lives. The writers share how the unknown is frightening, often more so than facing a terminal diagnosis. They share the emotional rollercoaster of treatments and remissions, and the numb shock one experiences when they hear the words, "There's nothing more we can do."

The stories explain how the profound grief is mitigated not by time, but by immersion into that hellish emotion. They also reveal how gratitude helps them to navigate this path daily.

In 2000, my aunt Wanda died at age sixty-four, nearly thirty years after her diagnosis. Against the odds, she outlasted the prognosis and outlived every one of those eight oncology specialists. Over twenty-five surgeries and treatments were endured, each designed to stabilize her through those years, and our family was grateful for every day.

Life is never predictable. We constantly need to shift our balance in response to events that flow and shape each day. The collection of stories within these pages provide comfort and hope, and serve as a gentle reminder that we too can—and will—survive loss by cancer.

DANA BROTHERS, B.S.
Outreach and Education Program Manager
Hospice of the Northwest
DBrothers@hospicenw.org

BY LYNDA CHELDELIN FELL

Preface

Cancer. It's a terrible word that strikes fear deep in the heart. From the very moment the diagnosis is delivered, our world pivots in unimaginable ways.

In 2006, our family joined the ranks of millions who found their lives invaded by cancer. It struck the baby of our family, my thirty-six-year-old sister Stacy. A mother of two little girls, she enjoyed a healthy lifestyle that included growing and selling organic vegetables at a local farmers market. Eschewing all chemicals, she had favored holistic remedies for years, making her the least likely victim in our family.

In spring 2006, Stacy, her husband, and their two girls moved into a stately six-bedroom home. About that same time, Stacy noticed a lump in her left armpit. She chalked it up to the strains of moving into a larger home and ignored it for the next eight months.

Come that November, the lump was still there and Stacy noticed strange sensations in the arm. She finally went to see her naturopath.

Alarmed, the naturopath was suspicious of something sinister and immediately sent Stacy for a battery of tests. The devastating results arrived the day before Thanksgiving. Stacy had stage IV breast cancer with metastases to her bones.

As a young woman with two little girls, doctors formulated a potent treatment plan. Stacy was scheduled for immediate surgery with plans for chemotherapy and radiation. But preop bloodwork revealed a second shock—Stacy was pregnant. And the cancer was feeding on the hormones that were vital to the baby.

Finding her case beyond his scope, the local oncologist sent Stacy to Seattle. Because the pregnancy hormones were the cancer's food source, the panel of doctors unequivocally felt that Stacy's best chance for survival depended upon immediate termination of the pregnancy followed by aggressive treatment. The doctors told her it was her only hope. The cancer was too advanced, and there was no time to waste: it was either Stacy's life, or the baby. They couldn't save both.

Stacy was known for her devout faith. And stubbornness. Despite pressure from the best oncologists in the state, she refused to terminate the unexpected pregnancy. Doctors wanted to know why.

"I wouldn't give up my other two children, I'm not giving up this one. So you need to figure out a plan B," was Stacy's reply.

My family was devastated. And scared. But Stacy refused to consider any other option.

An older, less effective chemotherapy deemed safer for the developing baby was planned. Nicknamed Red Death, the goal was to slow the cancer and buy time until the baby could be born. Stacy began treatment immediately but after five rounds of Red Death, the baby started showing signs of distress. Treatment had to stop.

Things went from bad to worse. An MRI showed the cancer had spread to Stacy's spine, and was marching downward. At thirty-two weeks gestation, the unborn baby needed to be delivered before cancer reached the womb.

Less than forty-eight hours later, Jazmine Stacy Roorda was born. Weighing less than four pounds and lacking sucking and swallowing reflexes that hadn't yet developed, she was otherwise perfect.

With the pregnancy behind her, two young daughters at home, and a preemie in NICU, Stacy now faced cancer treatment head on.

What happened next is what some might call a miracle: the treatment designed to buy Stacy a bit more time instead brought the cancer to a standstill. And it hasn't budged since.

My sister's journey with cancer is now nearly twelve years old. Her premature daughter is now a spunky eleven year-old with silky strawberry-blonde hair. But with metastases to Stacy's bones, she'll never be considered in remission. She has long outlived her gloom-and-doom prognosis, but the future remains unwritten.

Unless a cure is found soon, at some point Stacy's cancer will spread to her vital organs. When it does, I will hold this book in my hands and draw strength from the written words. As poignant as these stories are, each is an important reminder that the journey through losing a loved one to cancer is survivable. Filled with understanding and compassion, the stories will serve as my life raft in the storm and give me hope that if these writers survived, I will too. And that is what this book is all about.

Wishing you healing and hope from the Grief Diaries village.

Warm regards,

Lynda Cheldelin Fell

Creator, Grief Diaries
www.LyndaFell.com

CHAPTER ONE

The Beginning

And the idea of just wandering off to a cafe with
a notebook and writing and seeing where that
takes me for a while is just bliss. -J. K. ROWLING

Every story starts at the beginning, and so do our journeys. What was life like before that pivotal moment when it became divided by before and after?

*

JANICE DEL VECCHIO

Janice lost her husband Stephen to bile duct cancer in 2006 at age 47, and her second husband John to pancreatic cancer in 2013 at age 55

I've been widowed twice, once when I was forty-four and again at age fifty-two. Although both experiences had similar circumstances, each death had their own unique differences.

I was forty-two when my first husband Steve was diagnosed with inoperable bile duct cancer. Steve had caught a horrific cold from me and couldn't seem to recover from it. He went to his doctor and was given antibiotics for bronchitis. He completed the antibiotics and was still very sick. He was given a stronger antibiotic and still had no improvement. His physician ordered a CBC and liver profile blood tests to help determine what was wrong. The liver profile tests came back showing higher than normal bilirubin. I was concerned but wasn't thinking cancer at this point. Steve was always the worst case scenario guy and immediately started thinking he had all kinds of diseases. I did my best to try to allay his fears and remain calm until the test was repeated. When the second round of labs showed his bilirubin was still high, a CT scan and ultrasound were ordered.

A few days later the doctor called and asked Steve to come in, and to bring his wife. We were very concerned but hoped that whatever was wrong would be fixable.

We drove in silence to the appointment. When we met the doctor, she said a mass was growing near Steve's liver and bile ducts. I immediately knew what was wrong because a family acquaintance had recently passed away from the same cancer. I just lost it and started to cry. Steve was shocked and immediately asked me to please try to calm down; he needed me to be strong and support him. I understood what he was saying, but explained I was just told that my husband of twenty years had an incurable cancer. How did he expect me respond? Life as I knew from that point would never be the same.

I was fifty-one when my second husband John was diagnosed with inoperable pancreatic cancer. We had been married six months but lived together for a year prior.

After work one night, John went to the gym to work out. He came home earlier than expected and said he felt lousy—he could barely finish his workout and felt like he was going to pass out. I told him to lie down for a bit to see if it passed. It subsided somewhat. John took a shower and we went to bed.

I urged John to call his doctor and make an appointment as soon as possible. He had an appointment within two days and asked me to go with him. He picked me up at work and we drove in silence to the appointment. While he was driving, I glanced over and noticed the whites of John's eyes were yellow. I felt physically ill but kept my composure and didn't tell him about his eyes. I prayed that it would be gallstones or curable hepatitis.

I went into the exam room with John and the doctor immediately noticed he was jaundiced. Blood tests and scans were ordered and revealed a tumor on the pancreas. We both broke down but tried to console each other. John apologized over and over that I again had to go through this. He always put other people's feelings ahead of his own. In that moment, I knew life had once again thrown another curve ball. I seriously doubted I could do this again.

*

CYNTHIA HORACEK
Cynthia's husband Don died from
rectal cancer in 2010 at age 57

Don had a chronic illness called Crohn's disease, or inflammatory bowel disease. Crohn's is a terrible condition affecting people in a variety of ways. Most are able to lead a relatively normal life, but some are disabled from an early age.

Crohn's can strike people as young as infancy, but usually strikes by the mid to late-twenties. Don was diagnosed at age twenty-five, just before he and I met. We knew each other only four months before we were married, knowing a good thing when we saw it. We have two daughters and now five grandchildren. Even with his chronic illness, we lived a good and full life, and I'd marry him all over again, even knowing what our future would hold. Don was a wonderful husband and father; I credit his parenting for the wonderful people our daughters are today.

Don had been ill, mostly with bleeding from his Crohn's disease. There is always bleeding with this illness, so we didn't consider it might be due to something else. But he continued to lose weight and his doctor decided to do a scope of Don's intestines. A piece of tissue came out when he removed the scope and he sent it pathology.

That night, the doctor called and asked to speak with Don, asking me to say on the extension.

"Don, you have cancer," he said bluntly.

First thing the next morning, we called the surgeon who had performed surgery on Don in the past. Head of the department at Cedars-Sinai Hospital in Los Angeles, he was the best colorectal surgeon in the area.

He wasn't able to remove the entire tumor but the lymph nodes they took from Don's groin were all negative, leading us to have hope that he would beat this. He was referred for radiation and then chemo.

All was going well until Don's liver enzymes became elevated and he had to stop chemo. The oncologist said all looked good; the tumor didn't appear to be growing or spreading.

Then the unthinkable happened. Don began bleeding into his ostomy bag. We went to the emergency room and he was admitted to the hospital. By the end of the week, a bone marrow biopsy showed the cancer had metastasized. He was given several days to a few weeks.

Our daughters and Don's brother came to join us in vigil by Don's bedside. The end came pretty fast, which was a blessing for Don but not for us. I told him it was okay to go, but all I wanted to say was, "Don't leave me!"

When Don was first diagnosed I told him he wasn't allowed to die. But when someone you love is dying, sometimes he or she needs permission to let go. Loving someone makes you want to help their passage be as easy as possible.

Neither Don nor I were religious people but on that last morning, Don kept reaching toward the ceiling. Suddenly, at the very end he said, "Well, I guess so," and took his last breath.

I know in my heart and gut that Don saw something only he could see. It made me question my entire belief system. I believe that we will be together again, in a better place.

*

MARGARET HUTSELL
Margaret's 77-year-old husband Tom
died from pancreatic cancer in 2016

It seems like yesterday, and it came without warning. It was the dreaded C word and it was presented to us, in the car, on the way home from the grocery store back in September 2015.

I was surprised, terrified, and full of questions at the diagnosis of Tom's pancreatic cancer. It had not appeared in any history of his family tree and he was an active, engaged husband, father, grandfather, and my world. This cancer is one of the worst in survival rate graphs. This cancer gets little funding and seems to be diagnosed more often and in younger people than ever before. What did we do wrong was the question that most frequently popped into our minds. Did we eat the wrong things? Drink one too many glasses of wine?

I remember asking a ton of questions, calling a multitude of family and friends, and praying—lots of praying.

I watched my husband of fifty-six years journey through fourteen months of weight loss, muscle loss, eating problems, and emergency room visits in the middle of the night. Always waiting for doctors, nurses, labs to be drawn, lab results to be given, chemo rooms, CAT scan waiting rooms, and huge parking garages that were always filled by the time I arrived!

I talked with doctors and technicians after biliary catheter and ascites drains were installed, changed, and removed, never really completely understanding all the medical terms used so freely. I panicked when sepsis was diagnosed and I was brought into his ICU room to find him intubated and unconscious with a fever of 104.5. I learned how to give belly injections to offset the blood clots found in his lungs late in the game. No one had mentioned this possibility or told us it was common due to the many months of chemo infusions. No one had warned me about this part of the journey.

I learned, very quickly, that plans and dreams can be made, but might not be part of God's plan for us. I learned how to cope with stress and fear and exhaustion. I learned how to share these feelings with my rock, my best friend in the whole wide world, the guy who always had my back, my counselor, my lover, and my constant companion.

We discussed death and dying over coffee and/or wine. We talked about what my life would be like when alone for the first time in seventy-seven years. We talked about where he wanted to be at the time of his death and who he wanted to see the last few weeks of getting to that end point. We did nothing we didn't want to do and saw no one we didn't want to see and talked, and talked, and talked. I prayed for a miracle and realized I was living a miracle, with Tom, every day we had after diagnosis. His pain was controlled, his appetite wasn't too bad throughout, his strength and compassion for the pain of those witnessing his decline was constant.

I had the honor to care for him and journey with him as his life ended. I miss him constantly and my life will never be the same again.

"Different" is difficult, "we" is now "me." I didn't ask for this to happen and prayed, always, that it wouldn't. I have forgotten who I am and finding out is tough.

Tom and I never asked, "Why us?" My bucket list was only to grow old with him. Many would say that seventy-seven was old and fifty-six years together was enough. I say there is never enough time, yet death is part of life and so it goes.

I attended two support groups after Tom's death and continue with a therapist weekly. I love to talk about Tom and relive memories of our life together with anyone who will listen. As I write this, it has been two years since Tom died. I continue to wear my wedding ring and actually had Tom's band soldered to mine and together, they are just one more symbol of my continued love for him.

I continue to cry though a little less each week. I am grateful for the life I have had, and feel blessed to have had Tom to share it with. As I move forward (and we all will) I am blessed to have the time to make strong my relationship with God.

*

LYNN JORDAAN
Lynn's 58-year-old husband Johan
died from esophageal cancer in 2014

Johan was feeling unwell, not sick, just low and very tired, he kept saying he felt as if he had swallowed an eraser. I eventually persuaded him to visit our family physician who sent him for stress tests and an electrocardiogram because he thought Johan may have a heart problem. The results came back that it was not a heart problem, so the physician decided that a colonoscopy and gastroscopy were the next tests to complete.

My world was on the verge of imploding. The specialist asked me to join him with my husband in a tiny little closet of a room, where he proceeded to blurt out that Johan had cancer of the esophagus. It was too far gone to turn it around and that Johan was to start getting his affairs in order. This was said in one sentence, with no stopping for air. With that, the specialist turned and left the room, while we sat in stunned silence.

I am still not sure how we left the room and joined my daughter who was in the waiting room and got to the car. She kept asking us if everything was okay but neither of us had the courage to answer her. It was on the way to the car that Johan told her, and there I was, now holding them both up in the middle of a busy parking lot.

*

GAIL MARCHESA
Gail's husband John died from
colon cancer in 2009 at age 55

My husband, John, began feeling tired and was losing weight. When he started having pain, he finally went to the doctor. They sent John for a colonoscopy and found a mass. Unfortunately it had already spread to his liver. He began chemotherapy, and for months it seemed to work but eventually it spread to his lungs. He decided he had had enough. He was in hospice for only ten days and then died.

John had a good sense of humor. In fact, the funeral director said he never had so much fun planning a memorial. John wanted to have the last word on that. He wanted his ashes in Wyoming, and said I didn't have to go, just have FedEx drop him over it. What a goof. He was diagnosed May 2008 and passed March 21, 2009.

*

HEATHER MCLAUGHLIN
Heather's 35-year-old husband Derek
died from colorectal cancer in 2013

Derek and I were married on June 18, 2005. It was a perfect day. As we settled into marriage, about six months down the line Derek started getting cramps and bad stomachaches. We ignored them and treated them for what they were.

Fast forward to beginning of summer 2006. Derek had been bleeding and finally decided to tell me, but I know it had been going on for at least a couple of months. Twice we went to the emergency room because he was in such severe pain. Twice, because Derek was only twenty-nine, they pushed him to the side saying, "It's just a fissure or a tear." Finally, the parent of one of my students was an internist. He examined Derek and initially said the same thing but ordered a colonoscopy just to be sure.

We were so sure it was nothing that I taught school that day while Derek's dad took him. And then he sent me a text.

"They are pretty sure it's cancer." It rocked our whole world.

From that point on we didn't have time to comprehend and barely had time to breathe. He was immediately sent to a doctor in Atlanta. From there, prep for chemo, prep for radiation and go.

Derek was twenty-nine at the time of his diagnosis, and I was twenty-six. We weren't that far into our marriage come August 2007, but cancer had invaded our life.

We learned that Derek's cancer was a high stage III (3C). A port was placed and then he started chemotherapy. Oh, the joys we had with ports. He had five ports in five and a half years.

Derek had chemo and radiation every day for five weeks. His parents got a suite for him so he could stay next to the hospital. His mom stayed with him during the week so I could continue to teach. Thursday afternoons I drove down to Atlanta. His mom and I would talk about the week and then she headed to our house to take care of the dogs. I took care of Derek on the weekends and tried to lift his spirits. Either late Sunday or very early Monday morning, his mom and I would switch again so I could teach the next week. We ended the chemo and radiation on Derek's birthday, October 12.

We had to leave a bit of time between the end of the treatment and the first surgery, which was scheduled for November. I remember it was cold in Atlanta. We drove Derek there and then waited. The doctor asked to see us, so Mom, Dad and I went back.

He said, "I don't think I got it all," or something like that. Derek didn't want a colostomy bag at that point, and taking out the lymph nodes would have done that. Regardless, I stopped listening because all I heard was that the doctor didn't get it all. I was beside myself. How could he not? It's his job! When we went back to the waiting area to sit with other family members, Mom and Dad sat down and consoled each other. I ended up going for a heated walk with one of Derek's aunts. I let out my anger. I came back, ready to help Derek face what he needed to face.

Early 2007, we went to Sloan-Kettering for another opinion. The doctors thought they could help. We went twice but then the surgeon died and no one else wanted our case. That ended Sloan-Kettering.

We seemed okay for a little while, better than okay. We started trying for a family, but we always knew the cancer could come back.

Derek started feeling bad again, I honestly don't remember when. We found a good colon doctor at the Cleveland clinic in Florida. He looked everything over and assured us he could do surgery and even keep Derek's colon intact, so no colostomy bag!

The surgery was set for June 2011. It took six-plus hours before the doctor came to see me. The rest of the family was eating so I was alone when the doctor said, "We got all the cancer, but..." I'm thinking to myself, but what?

"But your husband ended up with a colostomy bag." I'm dumbfounded.

"A permanent one?" I asked.

"Yes."

By this time the rest of the family had returned, so the doctor repeats it. I was scared and started crying. We thought this place was hope, and now our world was crushed.

When I was finally allowed to see Derek, he was heavily sedated. Every time he moved or groaned, they gave him more pain meds. He had bandages and didn't look like Derek. I sat quite far away from his bed because I was afraid to get near him, like I might hurt him. I was crying silent tears. At one point Derek looked at me and asked if it was permanent or temporary, and I told him we would talk about it later. That later conversation was a really hard one for us both.

Derek ended up getting infections and not healing well from the surgery. He was hospitalized in Florida for a month before he was released. We then spent close to two weeks in a hotel before he could finally fly home to Charlotte. His wound was still not healing well and then became infected again. In August we returned to the hospital in Charlotte. It was there when we learned Derek now had spots on his lungs. The cancer had spread.

It was back with aggression and had advanced to stage IV-B. Derek tried new chemo drugs and also tried Avastatin at one point which started to lower his cancer marker numbers. Finally! But then in May 2012, Derek had a massive heart attack. Chemo was stopped for six months and we learned the heart attack was caused by the chemo drugs.

We knew the cancer was waging a war inside Derek's body. He wanted to take me to Europe, and go see Top Gear, so in August we went to England. It was scary with all the pain meds that he was on and the amount of pain he was in. We were in a new country and my husband was deathly ill. To say I was a wreck was not stretching it, but I tried to keep it as cool as possible for Derek.

Derek had masses on his kidneys and bladder. He had spots on his lungs and an abdominal infection caused by the cancer spreading into the abdominal nerves. It was everywhere. We signed up for hospice care. Some of the nurses who came to help knew what they were doing, and some didn't. Some days I knew more about the machine running Derek's wound VAC than they did. At the end, we had an amazing nurse who did everything in her power to help Derek get as comfortable as possible.

Derek died fighting for his last breath at a hospice house in Huntersville, North Carolina, on January 31, 2013.

*

SUE NOVA
Sue's husband Dana died from
lung cancer in 2012 at age 46

In 2009, my husband's doctor called and said his latest CT scan showed a small spot on his lung. We were getting ready to move across the country. We decided that as soon as we got settled, my husband would go see a doctor and get this figured out.

A couple weeks later we found ourselves sitting in the office of a thoracic surgeon who was describing the wedge resection surgery that he planned to perform. Turns out that Spot was too small to biopsy so they planned to remove him completely. While my husband was still on the operating table, Spot would be sent to pathology to determine whether it was malignant.

Pathology returned the results: it was cancer. Stage IB. The surgeon said they got it all. Nothing was in my husband's lymph nodes. All should be well.

Recovery went slow, but well. A year passed and work sent us back to California. As a good patient, my husband followed up with his doctor every six months for CT scans and blood work.

Sometime in early 2011, his oncologist said another tumor had appeared, and this time the regiment of chemo followed by radiation would be how to treat it. My husband and I had pretty much figured he was free and clear. After having a huge surgery and clear scans only to find out Spot was back and he was pissed was like a kick in the head.

I did as much research as I could about the type of lung cancer he had and I will say that the news was not promising. The life expectancy was less than ten percent at five years. Lung cancer kills more people than any other cancer and yet is the least funded. How is that possible? Oh, yeah…the stigma.

My husband tolerated the first round of chemo pretty well and sailed through the radiation. He continued working and we went on living life. After a break, new scans were done and new tumors found, so a fresh round of a different chemo began which, as predicted, caused what was left of his hair to fall out or get very thin. The talk of surgery was on the table. Perhaps remove the whole lung, perhaps a lobe. My husband chose to get a second opinion from a renowned thoracic surgeon at a famous teaching hospital in Los Angeles. The surgeon did say that either surgery was possible, but before anything could be done, we needed new CT scans from head to toe. This had to be done to ensure the cancer had not spread to any other organs, thus making the surgery a moot point. Once a cancer has metastasized (spread), surgery is no longer an option.

The scans were done and the news wasn't what we had hoped. The lung tumors remained static but the cancer had spread and now there were ten or so small lesions scattered on his brain. How do you even wrap your head around news like this? What were the next steps? How can this possibly be our life?!

We went back to his primary oncologist and were presented with options that weren't really options at all. First was a chemo pill taken once daily for ten days. It may or may not work because it's not for this type of cancer. Whole brain radiation was the second option, because the tumors were too small for gamma knife or cryosurgery. Because the chemo was less harsh, so it seemed, it was the initial choice but if it didn't have any effect, then whole brain radiation would be next. Whole brain radiation is exactly what it sounds like—they radiate the whole brain. They made a mesh and plastic mask for his face, he laid on a table, the mask was placed over his face and bolted to the table, and he was zapped every day for twenty-one days. If I knew then what I know now, whole brain radiation would not have been an option!

Through all of this my husband put on a brave face for me, his coworkers, and family. He never, to me, questioned why this was happening to him. I could tell, though, that he was tired. He was losing weight, his spirits flagged, and his temper grew short. Who could blame him? Certainly not me.

After the radiation, there was a break of all treatment for a couple of months. That made my husband nervous because, to him, if no treatment was happening, the cancer was growing.

The following months were filled with new chemo treatments, which didn't seem to help—now there were random tumors growing on his abdomen walls. A tumor growing on his jaw was pressing on a nerve and caused him unbearable pain.

In November 2011, his oncologist told him about a clinical trial. He was qualified and could start immediately. The trial showed much promise, though sadly not for him. The side effect of this drug was acne-like pustules on his face, head, and back. This man, my rock, never complained, even as he suffered.

The trial was stopped because the tumors continued to grow. He woke up one morning with the right side of his face paralyzed. The tumor on his jaw had finally constricted the nerve completely. Initially we thought it was Bell's palsy but we were wrong...again.

February 2012, was my husband's first hospitalization. He was lying in bed and told me his chest felt heavy like someone was sitting on it. Which indicated to me either blood clot or collapsed lung. Off we went to the emergency room. He was admitted and yes, it was a blood clot. He was then put on blood thinners that required him to self-administer an injection, daily, to his abdomen.

In March 2012, he woke me up and said he couldn't breathe. Off to the hospital we go. This time, because the tumor has grown so big, it's blocking the bronchus. I ask the attending about the next step. She says long-term antibiotics to ward off infection since the lung will basically be dying inside him.

They did another CT. They give me the results and I read them: the tumors have all grown rapidly. To further shatter my world, there are lesions all over his brain. Again. I tell my husband and we are determined, still, to kick this cancer's butt!

A few days later, he's discharged from the hospital. I loaded him and his ever present oxygen bottle into the car and we went to see his oncologist, who said we can do another round of chemo. Since I am aware only one chemo passes through the blood/brain barrier, I ask if the new chemo will work on the lesions on his brain. The doctor looks at me very confused, and turns to continue reading the report. While he was reading, I saw his posture slump and his whole demeanor changed. He turned back to us and said that more chemo would only prolong the inevitable, but we could still do it. My husband, being the trouper that he was, said he was ready to go and that he was, finally, willing to get a port installed. Keep in mind, he was probably weighing in at one hundred forty pounds by this time.

We come home and continue to live. He's getting weaker, unable to walk unassisted. He's forgetful. The tumor on his jaw is still growing and he's in a lot of pain. I learn a lot about the hard work of being a full-time caretaker and am only sleeping a few hours a day. He gets very agitated if I am not home with him.

Beginning of May 2012, he went to have a chemo treatment. He's sick, weak, in pain, and the nurses are unable to find a vein.

That was the day we have the conversation. I told him he can quit treatment and just come home with me. He asks if I'm okay with that. Oh, honey, how could I not be? We started hospice a day or so later.

My beloved husband died quietly and surrounded by love at 9:44 a.m. on May 29, 2012.

*

SHERYL POCHEL
Sheryl's husband Brian died from
pancreatic cancer in 2011 at age 43

Brian was diagnosed with pancreatic cancer in February 2006, at the age of thirty-eight. At the time, I was thirty-six and our children were six, four, two, and ten months old. We were given little to no hope that he would survive. The oncologist's prognosis was, "A year, probably not two."

For months prior to his diagnosis, Brian hadn't been feeling well after he ate. It wasn't anything specific, just overall didn't feel good. I remember in November 2005, we were going to dinner at our favorite restaurant to celebrate our birthdays, which were three days apart. He said, "I don't even want to go." When I asked why, he said, "I just don't feel good after I eat." It was the first time he had really said anything, though once we knew he had cancer I can look back and remember other things he said and activities he missed with our family because his stomach was upset.

I asked him at that point if he needed to go see a doctor, his answer was no, he was sure he was fine. In reality, (and he only said this one time, but boy has it stuck with me) he thought he was having gallbladder issues, and would have to have his gallbladder removed. We had plans that year to visit his dad and stepmom for Christmas and he didn't want to go to the doctor because he didn't want to ruin our vacation. How I wish I had pushed him to go.

He first went to the doctor in January 2006. They thought it was acid reflux and prescribed Prilosec and said to call back in two weeks. He took one of the pills, knew that wasn't it and didn't take any more, but waited two weeks before going back to the doctor. They started doing more tests, but because of his age they didn't do the right ones. No one was even thinking pancreatic cancer. He didn't smoke, drink, do drugs. He was an athlete, a chiropractor and lived a heathy lifestyle. No family history of cancer. Yet, he was diagnosed with pancreatic cancer on February 27, 2006. It was devastating.

Brian survived well past his prognosis of "a year, probably not two." In fact, he lived for five and a half years after his diagnosis, and while there were some very rough times, most of it was a good quality life. Our kids all had the chance to know him and have concrete memories of him. He passed away on September 3, 2011, while I laid by his side, holding him. In the end, in that moment, it was just us, even though the room was full of family.

There is not a day that goes by that I don't think of him and miss him with all of my being. Moving forward has been hard. Being an only parent is definitely a challenge. My family and friends have kept me sane and I will be forever thankful that they have stayed by my side through all of this. Being widowed takes a strength from within that you don't even know exists until you are faced with no other choice. Six years after his death I am in a good place. I'm happy, I'm moving forward with my life, and that is a good thing.

*

KATHIE SCOTT
Kathie's 57-year-old husband Jim
died from prostate cancer in 2009

My husband was diagnosed with stage IV prostate cancer in 2005. Several years prior, he had an infection that cleared with antibiotics and nothing was ever mentioned about follow up or checking on PSA levels. I'm not sure how long he had symptoms as he had been through a heart attack and bypass surgery just four years earlier, so I think he was reluctant to see a doctor. When the symptoms indicated he had no choice but to see a doctor, off he went to see his primary physician who didn't see any urgency. Only after my husband suggested it, he was referred to a urologist but the appointment was scheduled for two months out.

In my research, his symptoms clearly indicated something serious and my advocacy mode kicked in. I phoned the urologist in tears, begging for an earlier appointment and this fine doctor immediately obliged. Within a few days the diagnosis had been delivered and our horrible journey through cancer began.

For the first few months, my husband had a periodic injection to lower his testosterone, and his numbers dropped for a few months but then started to climb. Upon further testing, chemotherapy was started.

The initial diagnosis indicated the cancer had spread to his bones and lymph nodes in the groin, but doctors agreed that no surgery was going to arrest it. His only treatment was radiation and chemotherapy.

From 2006 until his death in 2009, he was on this regiment. The cancer continued to spread to more areas of the body including the brain, a bone around one eye, his ribs, and hips. The doctors were all surprised the cancer had spread to his brain; it wasn't the typical path for prostate cancer. Regardless of what it should or shouldn't do, it had gone rogue. The headaches and double vision told us it was serious, so the next step was brain surgery.

My husband had a remarkable attitude about everything related to his illness. He accepted that he had to fight like he had never done before, and according to his doctors and nurses, he was the perfect patient with an engaging smile and sense of humor.

After two years of fighting and treatments, he could no longer work. He retired and tried to make the best of this free time that had been forced on him. The brain tumor appeared once more but was "successfully" treated with gamma knife surgery. By 2007, he was constantly on oxygen as the radiation to treat tumors on his ribs had damaged his lungs—one example where the treatment is often as bad as the disease.

We were high school sweethearts. For many years of our married life he had been in a bar band, because a world without music wasn't something he wanted to be part of. His taste in music was wide but the little band allowed him to play his drums and guitar on a regular basis. The guitar became the instrument of choice when the drums became too physically taxing. Many weekends through his illness he played with his oxygen tank part of the equipment. To say he had the best of friends would be an understatement.

In early 2008, he developed multiple blood clots in his lungs. We were in the emergency room, unsure of the diagnosis at that point. The doctor told him, "If I had what you have, I would go home, take my medicine, and wait to die." We were having none of that, so on went the ventilator and he spent a month recovering in the hospital.

He came home after six weeks but was unable to walk due to his bed confinement. We were blessed with a physical therapist who had him walking again in short order. He remained quite confined because no matter how high the oxygen level went, it couldn't overcome the damaged lungs. Even so, one week out of the hospital and rehab and he was playing his beloved music at a Relay For Life event!

For the better part of our life together, we had a dog in the house but were without one when the cancer was diagnosed. From the beginning we knew Jim's cancer would probably, at best, give him five or so years. We toyed with getting a dog but let cancer make the decision not to because it was one more thing to be responsible for.

In July 2009, since Jim was pretty much confined to the house all day alone, I decided his cancer was not going to win this one. Little Zoe, a Maltese-Yorkie mix, came into our lives and it was one of the best things in this mess. She and Jim became fast friends and even though she was only eight weeks old, she was in tune to her new dad's needs. He slept, she slept, and what should have been a high energy little dog was as quiet and loving as a big old lab. Little Zoe is now eight years old and her personality hasn't changed at all. She took on her dad's gentle demeanor for sure.

In October 2009, the first stroke reared its ugly head. Although mild, it was a worrisome milestone. A month later the second one hit and the only hint was that Jim's sentences weren't quite right during a phone conversation with his brother. I did a little triage and decided he needed to be checked. The emergency room doctor confirmed that Jim had probably had multiple small strokes and was admitted for further testing. Somewhere between the emergency room and the upper floor, he forgot who I was. When the nurse asked him who I was, he had no idea.

To be married for thirty-seven years and suddenly your husband has no idea who you are is beyond painful.

We spent a week in the hospital and finally the neurosurgeon told me I should look at taking Jim home under hospice care. There was nothing to be done but wait for the inevitable. I brought him home on Monday morning and he was gone Tuesday evening, surrounded by the people he loved most.

His illness had taken a sudden turn and it was as if Jim had no fight left in him. In discussing this with his doctor, her only conclusion was that the stroke had caused Jim to forget that he needed to fight. I understand that is probably not the case, but it was as if he just gave up and told the cancer to do what it wanted.

Like everyone who has walked this path, I feel like there were so many things I should have done differently. I did not want to discuss some very important things because, to me, that was a sign of giving up hope, and that was not going to happen. In retrospect, I wish I had been more realistic and accepting of the situation, yet I simply could not have those difficult conversations.

Five years after Jim died, I met a lovely man, also named Jim, and we have developed a terrific, loving relationship. It cannot compare to my marriage and the love is not as deep, but it's comforting knowing that once again I have someone to love and who loves me. Second loves and older loves are so very different from the young ones who have a thirty-seven-year history.

Widowhood is certainly not something I recommend and yet I've met many lovely people along the journey and we've managed to support and hold each other up when we are at our lowest.

*

STEVE SHARP
Steve's 51-year-old wife Carolyn
died from melanoma in 2014

Haven't I been here before? I remember standing on the beach in St. Augustine, Florida, when it finally hit me: I was now a "me" and no longer part of a "we."

Everywhere I looked, couples were doing things together and yet my companion was gone. I felt the loneliness of not fitting in any longer. Perhaps you may be able to identify with my story. I've been widowed twice. My first wife, Jean, had three children. We were married for eighteen years before she died of congestive heart failure from an autoimmune disease. My second wife, Carolyn, and I were married for fourteen years before she died from melanoma cancer after being diagnosed six and a half years earlier.

I honestly felt as though I'd won the lottery from hell twice! After Jean died, I was a single parent to our children ages seventeen, fifteen, and twelve. It was like I was living a nightmare and if I could only wake up, my life would magically return to normal. Do you know what it feels like to be trapped in a deep, dark hole? Out of desperation, I got my kids and myself into therapy before joining a spiritual-based support group. In time, I saw light shine through the darkness and began to think life could be good.

When I began to date again it was a disaster. The first few women I dated were divorcées. They seemed angry and unsure whether they had ever loved their spouses. As a widower, I had never stopped loving my wife. I couldn't relate to their previous marriages and they couldn't relate to mine. It was not a good experience.

Eventually, I joined an online dating group called Singles with Scruples and met my second wife, Carolyn. It was so good having someone to talk to who shared my experience of losing a spouse. We met in person at a Young Widowers Group in Virginia Beach, and began dating in early 2000. It was wonderful dating someone who understood me so well because of the shared loss of our spouses and both having walked through grief.

We fell in love and married that July. She brought her two kids, ages four and nine, into our marriage and I brought my three. Life was sweet again and we shared many experiences together: the marriages of our older children, family holidays, birth of four grandchildren, as well as traveling to many beautiful places. We were there for each other in the good and bad times of life. Carolyn's solid support helped me get through my parents' deaths. We understood that even in the happiest of occasions one could still be a little sad because our deceased spouse wasn't there to experience the joyous moment.

When Carolyn and I married, I naïvely thought I had earned an immunity badge that would prevent me from losing another spouse before I was old and gray. Surely God wouldn't take another wife from me. Well, I was wrong. Carolyn was diagnosed with skin cancer in February 2007. She began treatment, the cancer seemed to disappear, and we shared six and a half years free of worry. Sadly, the cancer returned—this time in her lymph nodes.

Carolyn was upbeat and expected to be back at work after a brief recovery. A high school chemistry teacher, she absolutely loved the young people she mentored. During surgery to remove the cancerous lymph nodes, however, they discovered more cancer in her stomach. She started a new drug called Zelboraf that eradicated the cancer in her stomach. We thought we were lucky and beat the cancer!

We went away to celebrate over Memorial weekend. On Sunday, when Carolyn woke up, she was having difficulty walking. Of course we were scared, and made a quick trip home to the emergency room. After a CAT scan, the doctor said, "You have interesting things in your brain." Not what we wanted to hear. A follow up MRI confirmed our worst fears. A number of large tumors were growing in her head.

The neurosurgeon who gave us the news said that time was short, probably only four months, and advised us to make the most of our remaining time together. Unfortunately, Carolyn weakened quickly and was hospitalized a number of times. She became progressively worse and there was nothing I could do about it. She struggled with memory, mood swings, pain, and grew weaker before my very eyes.

In October, when we learned she only had two weeks left, I tried to get her into hospice so she could be at home, but the situation was too difficult to manage and she died in a hospital.

Again, I faced the despair of losing someone I couldn't imagine living without. It's true you never get over losing a spouse. After Carolyn died, I also relived losing my first wife, Jean. Can you imagine trying to tread water carrying not one heavy stone, but two? I outlived two wonderful women who had so much to live for in this world. Jean was a dedicated NICU nurse and Lamaze instructor, and Carolyn was an innovative high school chemistry teacher who had such a positive impact on the lives of so many students.

I suffered survivor's guilt and questioned why I was still alive. The answer became obvious: our kids. I was the surviving parent to five kids. My youngest, a college freshman, came home one weekend in tears because she had to fill out a form that considered her to be an orphan since both her birth dad and mom had passed away.

There is a saying that time heals, but I believe that is only true if you are honest with yourself and work hard at it. So, what got me through another significant loss? Many things. We were very blessed to have a great group of friends who supported us through Carolyn's fight with cancer. They are still there for me today. Next, I joined a local hospice surviving spouse group who met twice a month. It was led by widows and widowers who absolutely got what I was going through.

I also joined an online support group: Widowed Village, which was where I could vent and learn from other grief journeys. Through this website I learned about Camp Widow. It sounded like it was just what I needed to help with my recovery. In retrospect, it was the hardest thing for me to do, but was also the best thing I did. I made the decision to drive to Camp Widow in Tampa from Virginia only four months after Carolyn died. The road trip proved to be a special time to be by myself and think.

Being at Camp Widow was a very special experience. The classes, conversations, and presentations seemed to talk directly to me. I was not alone. In fact, the experience was so positive, I made the decision to go a second time sixteen months later.

Michele Hernandez said there was a special quality that drew another person to us and that we didn't lose that quality when our spouse died. She said it was okay to forgive myself for surviving. Every Tuesday, I remembered Carolyn dying and loyally tried to hold onto the memory. Over time, Michele explained that the memory would become less painful though it didn't mean you loved them any less. I needed to hear that.

Another thing that helped me to heal was volunteering to lead a grief support group. It not only serves as an opportunity to remember what I went through and how I have become whole again, but as a way to be there for others in the hope that they may also recover and find happiness again. It helped me to see something positive come out of my tragedy. It happened to me and it can also happen to you.

*

AUDRA THEROUX
Audra's father died from
esophageal cancer in 2014

It is important to realize one thing about my father before I even begin to tell his story. My father was a Marine through and through. It was almost impossible to know when he was having pain because Marines are taught to "laugh in the face of pain." So by the time we realized my father was having symptoms, they were noticeable to others and hard to ignore. The first thing I noticed is that my father was burping a lot. He had also started to lose weight. In the past, I had had a few ulcers and had the exact same symptoms, so I thought for sure he had an ulcer. My father hated doctors and, of course, put off going. He was planning a trip in October to visit his mother in South Carolina and, after some nagging, agreed to go when he returned.

The trip to visit my grandmother took an unexpected turn. She fell ill and my father ended up having to stay longer. He was there for a month, and during that time, she passed away. This, of course, meant he did not see the doctor. He decided he would see the doctor after her funeral on December 26.

Come January, he had an appointment to see a gastroenterologist. He was then scheduled for an endoscopy so the doctor could look at his esophagus and stomach. It was scheduled for February 6, 2014. I will always remember the date. It was two days before my birthday, and the day before I was due to leave for vacation.

While waiting for the test, my father's symptoms seemed to get worse. He was having trouble swallowing food. He blamed the dry hospital air he experienced when he was with my grandmother. At the time, it never occurred to me that it was anything other than an ulcer. I only knew what I saw. My dad was not one to complain. All through his entire cancer journey, he never complained. So I had to judge what was happening by what I witnessed myself. I fully expected him to have an ulcer that could be treated and forgotten.

On February 6, I wasn't feeling well so my mother took my dad for the endoscopy. For the rest of my life, I'll never forget getting the news that Dad didn't have an ulcer. He was walking up the stairs after his test. I was sitting on the couch and asked him, "How'd the test go?"

He said, "I have a tumor," and walked into the kitchen.

He said it in the same way he would have said it was raining—like it was nothing. I honestly felt like my world was crashing down. I think in most people's mind the word tumor equates to cancer. At that time, we wouldn't have the biopsy results for another week or two, but in my mind, I just knew. I'm pretty sure he did, too. So, two days before my fortieth birthday, I unofficially learned my dad had cancer.

My dad seemed to handle the news well. He told us to go on our vacation as planned. There was nothing to be done until the biopsy results were back, and by then we'd be home. So that was what we did after a lot of urging from him.

Once the biopsy results confirmed the tumor was cancer of the esophagus, everything sprang into action fast. I researched the best doctors and got a referral for him to be seen in Massachusetts. We live in New Hampshire on the border and got him in pretty fast. Our first appointment was with a surgeon. She basically told us that his tumor was inoperable at that time, and referred him to an oncologis.

Everything moved fast and, with that, I have no complaints. In looking back, the only thing I wish we had done differently was to get him seen immediately when his symptoms first started. But due to my grandmother's health and my father's own stubbornness, I don't see how I could've changed things. I've replayed the scenario a million times and wonder if the end result could have been different. Knowing what I know now about esophageal cancer, it probably wouldn't have changed anything. But that doesn't stop me from wishing I had pushed harder for him to go to the doctor sooner.

*

STEPHANIE VANDERVALK
Stephanie's husband Rob died from
osteosarcoma in 2016 at age 24

I met my best friend, first love, soulmate, and husband in high school in September 2009. I was in grade eleven at the time and Rob was completing courses to get into Sheridan College for photography. We were in an art class for stained glass and sat across from each other at the working table. He was the older rebellious guy in the class and I was the goodie two-shoes. Somehow I managed to survive his endless teasing on the matter.

After some conversation, I found out that he had moved into my childhood home just a few months prior. It was as if I had never left. He felt like home to me. He managed to sweep me off my feet. I was told months before he died that he turned to his friend in stained glass class one day and said, "I'm going to marry her."

We dated for two years and lived out every Ryan Gosling movie you could think of before Rob was diagnosed with osteosarcoma in April 2012. What started out as knee pain turned into something no

33

twenty-one-year-old could ever imagine. Rob had osteosarcoma in his knee, the same type of cancer as Terry Fox.

He went through chemotherapy and a knee replacement that summer and we could both agree it was the longest and toughest six months of our lives. Rob always made the most of it, and we still had Friday night date nights every week.

Following the knee replacement, Rob was in remission. We were told there was a fifty percent chance this type of cancer could appear in his lungs, however Rob never let that hold him back. He pursued his career as a still life photographer working in Toronto.

In May 2013, we received news that the cancer had reached Rob's lungs. Chemotherapy and a lung resection later, the cancer was gone. We continued to live our lives and have hope that every scan would be clear. Rob refused to live every day with that thought hanging over his head. We would get lost in our days together and forget all reality. That was one of our favorite things. In looking back, I think that was how we coped.

A few months later, the cancer returned to Rob's lungs and had also spread to his kidney. More chemo, more surgeries. We wanted to make the most out of the situation, so prior to treatment we packed our bags and headed to Whistler, British Columbia. Rob wasn't going down without a fight. He knew his life was going to be short, so he insisted he follow out every dream he had. Riding the mountains in Whistler was one of the many things crossed off Rob's bucket list.

A few months later, we received another bout of bad news—the cancer had reached Rob's brain. He was shattered yet never showed defeat. He underwent what was supposed to be routine brain surgery, but woke up paralyzed on his left side. I've never seen someone with more perseverance, optimism, and dedication. Rob was determined to walk and get back on a bike, and he did.

During this time, Rob was still receiving treatment for his lungs. When told his cancer was no longer responding to chemotherapy, it was decided he would start a new experimental drug. He kept up his optimism.

Through all of this our relationship never faltered. Although we spent most of our time in hospitals, my love for him only grew more each day. He was my gift of love and joy and in August 2015, Rob asked me to be his wife. We planned our wedding for summer 2018, after I had graduated from nursing school. We were going to have three children and live in the country. We had big dreams for a life together, and couldn't have been more excited.

Three days later our world came crashing down. The cancer was in Rob's brain, and the experimental drug for the lungs was no longer effective. We were broken, yet it didn't stop us. With help from family and friends, we married two months later on October 12, 2015. It was a beautiful, sunny day, and like a fairytale. I promised Rob that in the pressures of the present and the uncertainties of the future, I would be there for him. He promised me his never-ending love, and said I would never be alone, no matter how far away he is. How perfect.

A week later Rob was admitted to the palliative floor. The cancer had spread to his liver and spine. Moving to hospice was now part of the conversation. On November 30, 2015, Rob moved to Lisaard House in Cambridge, Ontario, where he lived the rest of his life with gratitude in his heart. He died January 15, 2016.

Rob was the most courageous, stubborn, and thoughtful man I have ever known. I am proud to have been his wife, even if it was only for three months. I wouldn't change the last seven years for anything. Rob taught me a new definition of strength. He taught me to live every day like it's your last, and to never give up on your dreams. There are no guarantees in this life. Be happy. Be bold. Laugh. I know Rob is riding the mountains up in heaven, and walks alongside us every day. Rest in peace my darling babe. This one is for you.

*

DIANNE WEST
Dianne's husband Vern died from
multiple myeloma in 2010 at age 69

Life was good in 2006. I had a demanding job I loved; Vern had retired from teaching and was working as the guest services manager for a sports and entertainment arena in Las Vegas. We were looking forward to returning to Maui in June to celebrate our thirty-seventh wedding anniversary. And then cancer arrived.

Vern had back issues that flared from time to time, so we weren't initially alarmed when the pain began early in 2006. However, when Vern got to the point when he could barely walk, I convinced him to see a doctor. A CT scan didn't show anything, so he was sent for physical therapy. That didn't help and, in fact, made it much worse. We reached out again to his primary physician and begged him to get insurance approval for an MRI to figure out what was going on. We weren't home too long after the procedure when his doctor called.

"My God, man, you have a tumor on your spine."

I can still hear those words in the doctor's southern drawl, and can still see the look on my husband's face. An appointment had been scheduled for us to see another doctor early the next morning. That was a hard night. Vern wasn't one to share his feelings in great detail, and I talk to think. I don't think either of us slept.

Vern was in great pain, so it was very difficult getting him out of bed and into the car the next morning. Once we arrived, I got him into a wheelchair and we were taken to a very small room. Vern in a wheelchair, me on a stool, and the doctor showing us MRI scans. The tumor. The hot spots. Spinal compression fractures. So many lytic lesions. Multiple myeloma. Cancer. Metastasized. Not a good prognosis.

The doctor felt it was important to do surgery the next day, so we were told to go straight to the hospital. We were overwhelmed with this news. Numb. The hospital was just two miles away but I didn't drive there immediately. It was a hot day in May, so I found a shaded residential street and pulled over to the curb. We sat in silence for a few minutes, just holding hands. And then I asked if we should see another doctor, get a second opinion, find other options. Vern said no. He just wanted this thing removed as quickly as possible.

And so it began. Our cancer journey.

Their immediate focus was removing the tumor and stabilizing the spine so Vern wouldn't be paralyzed. Surgery was scheduled for the following afternoon, but first there were more labs, another more extensive MRI, lots of tests and scans. After over four hours in surgery, the tumor was gone and I was hopeful that the titanium cage around his spine would allow Vern to walk again. At that point I really hadn't started to think about dealing with the cancer diagnosis.

Vern appeared to be making progress and was moved out of ICU, but two days after surgery something was very wrong. Vern's coloring was off and his skin felt cold and clammy. He complained of heaviness in his chest and said something wasn't right. I went out to get the nurse but she couldn't come immediately, so I returned and went to the opposite side of Vern's bed so the nurse could have easy access to him when she arrived. That's when I saw the bright red blood flowing into his chest tube bag. I ran back to the nurse and within seconds his room filled with staff. His blood pressure had dropped dangerously and they pushed four bags of blood into him before taking him to the OR.

That was a rough day. The surgeon came out afterward and told me Vern had gone into cardiac arrest but they were able to revive him with manual manipulation and paddles. Then he said Vern had been given four units of the wrong blood. I was grateful for his honesty but concerned about the impact since Vern had a blood cancer. The doctor contacted several experts about this and felt confident there would not be a lasting impact. I prayed he was right.

Vern was on a ventilator in ICU and looked far worse than he had after the initial surgery. But he was alive and I was grateful. Two weeks later he was moved to a rehab facility to regain his ability to walk; he wouldn't make it home for another ten weeks.

Three weeks of rehab and then a GI bleed sent Vern back to the hospital for a week. He returned to rehab and then came down with pneumonia, had a pulmonary embolism, and needed to start chemo which sent him back to the hospital for three weeks. This became our life for the next five months. In and out of the hospital, rehab, or a long-term acute care facility.

They told us that chemo and radiation would hopefully give Vern eighteen months. We got over four years, but they were very, very hard years. Lots of infections and blood transfusions. A colostomy. Kidney failure and dialysis. Even a life-threatening abdominal aortic pseudoaneurysm caused by a screw in the titanium cage. He had excellent medical care; he had horrible medical care.

I spent every waking moment doing everything in my power to keep Vern positive, to care for him, and to ease his pain. I learned to take care of a colostomy bag and a PICC line, to hang IVs at home, and give him shots in his belly. I researched possible treatments and served as his advocate with the many doctors, nurses, and medical staff. I got him to the dialysis center three mornings a week, administered meds and kept track of it all, and took him for weekly chemo. He went through so much. And then there was nothing more they could do to him. Or for him.

His final days were spent at Nathan Adelson Hospice. No more pricks and prods or waking him up for rounds. He was peaceful. And those final four days were a gift. He spoke very little the first two days and then was silent, but I have no doubt at all that he heard my words. When the death rattle arrived, I gently slid into his bed, held him close and spoke to him until he slipped away hours later.

My life was forever changed. I was fifty-nine years old and had never lived alone in my entire life. I grieved the loss of my love, and I even grieved the loss of being his caregiver.

I returned to work immediately. I needed the normalcy. I cried on the way into work, fixed my makeup in the parking lot, and walked through the gate as I had done before I was widowed. I acted normal all week long and crashed on the weekends. I worked four ten-hour shifts, so when I arrived home at 7 p.m. on Thursdays, I put on my pajamas, closed the blinds, and did not step outside, answer the phone or door all weekend long. I did not take good care of myself or my home. But during those forty-plus hours on the job, and my positive Facebook and Widowed Village posts, no one had a clue of how close to the edge I was actually living.

Eight years have now passed since I held Vern in my arms. Time has softened the pain but hasn't changed how much I miss him.

I've retired. I spend a lot of time volunteering. I've done some traveling. I've taken classes, started a little business. I'm living my life. And I'm doing my best to live it well to honor him, because I am who I am today because he loved me.

CHAPTER TWO

The Symptoms

When it rains, look for rainbows. When
it's dark, look for stars. -ANONYMOUS

Every journey through cancer begins at the starting gate—the moment when a one-worded diagnosis permanently alters every life path. What led up to that point? What signs could no longer be ignored?

*

CYNTHIA HORACEK
Cynthia's husband Don died from
rectal cancer in 2010 at age 57

The diagnosis was missed during the first few scopes and scans.

*

MARGARET HUTSELL
Margaret's 77-year-old husband Tom
died from pancreatic cancer in 2016

We had just returned from a weekend visit with our son and his family in Illinois, and Tom felt itchy from head to toe. We thought he might have stirred up an old allergy while away, and he took Benadryl. Little did we know that our lives would change on a dime once we followed up on a simple itch.

The Benadryl didn't help much. After a couple of sleepless nights and distracted days, I finally convinced my stoic and resolved husband of fifty-six years to seek professional help at a nearby urgency clinic that was lovely and professionally well-staffed. We arrived, waited to see a doctor and walked out an hour later with a diagnosis of hepatitis C. Blood work had been taken, and hands-on touching and feeling and prodding completed. The only thing suspicious was Tom's elevated bilirubin. The physician suggested we follow up with our primary care physician and we made an appointment for the next morning.

Dr. L gave Tom the once over and noticed a bit of jaundice. He ordered a CT for the next day, a Friday in mid-September 2015. Why didn't I see the jaundice? I'll never, ever know.

Friday morning was brisk and cool. Off we drove to a local clinic for the CT scan. We were told that results would be phoned to us the following Monday. Pleased the medical stuff was now done, off we drove to the grocery store, as per our normal routine.

*

LYNN JORDAAN
Lynn's 58-year-old husband Johan
died from esophageal cancer in 2014

Don had been ill for a few months before they found his cancer. With Crohn's disease (inflammatory bowel disease) there is almost always bleeding so we didn't think much about it. He continued to lose weight, and his blood pressure was too low and that made his doctor want to do another scope. So, there weren't many symptoms that were unusual. I think that might have made the diagnosis more of a shock.

*

GAIL MARCHESA
Gail's husband John died from
colon cancer in 2009 at age 55

I, for one, was mad. John was sick for a month before even making a doctor appointment. Then another two weeks before a colonoscopy. John took the news very matter-of-factly but you could tell he was shocked. A year prior, he had gotten sick and needed to vomit, I have to say it was all over and black. That's when I started bugging him to go to the doctor. He was very stubborn and chalked it up to getting older and goofy hours at work.

*

HEATHER MCLAUGHLIN
Heather's 35-year-old husband Derek
died from colorectal cancer in 2013

Before Derek was officially diagnosed we knew he was sick. He had been having some gastro issues before and being the type of people we are, we didn't like to go to the doctor. When Derek finally told me he was in a lot of pain during the summer 2006, he was bleeding from his rectum. We ended up being seen in the emergency room twice that summer, with both visits ending the same. "It is most likely a fissure or a tear. Go home, take some of these pain meds, and take a bath. It will clear up on its own." It wasn't until one of my student's parents, who was an internist, decided to see him, took things another step and asked for a colonoscopy as well. Honestly, Derek and I were so convinced that it was a fissure or a tear, that his dad took him. I got a text message from him while I was teaching, "they think it's cancer." It changed our life forever. We didn't believe it at first. We went and saw well known specialists in Atlanta, Georgia and they gave us the same diagnosis. We were rushed into pre op meetings and surgeries to set up a five-week intensive course chemotherapy and radiation to attack the cancer hard. It had attacked us hard, it was charted at a stage IIIB.

*

SUE NOVA
Sue's husband Dana died from
lung cancer in 2012 at age 46

Dana had none, I repeat, no signs or symptoms. His first dance with cancer was found completely by accident. He had an abdominal CT done for gastrointestinal issues in August 2008. For some reason, his doctor called him at the end of October and said there was a small spot on his lung that was something he should get checked out. We were preparing to move across the country from California to Illinois, and life literally stopped.

We spent time talking to trusted friends and his doctor. They assured us that Chicago had some of the best hospitals and doctors, and that we should go. So we did.

*

SHERYL POCHEL
Sheryl's husband Brian died from
pancreatic cancer in 2011 at age 43

Looking back, I remember that Brian started vocalizing his stomach problems eight months before he was diagnosed. We had just had our fourth baby and had outgrown our home. I found a house I wanted to put an offer on, but Brian was resistant. One Thursday in June 2005, we were taking our kids to a state park for the day. As we entered the park, we were talking about the house I wanted.

Brian sighed and said, "Fine, we'll put an offer in, but if I'm getting an ulcer I'm blaming you!"

The following month he missed the family fireworks. He thought he had eaten something that wasn't agreeing with him, and didn't want to leave home. In November, we were going to our favorite restaurant to celebrate our birthdays, which were three days apart. On our way there, Brian said, "I don't even want to go." I asked him why.

"Because I just don't feel good after I eat," he said.

I asked him if he needed to see a doctor. He said no, he was sure he was fine. He was chiropractor, so I didn't question him when it came to his health. I wish I had pushed harder.

After he was diagnosed, he said the reason he didn't want to see a doctor was because he thought it was his gallbladder and worried he was going to need to have it removed. He said he didn't want to ruin our trip to Alabama to spend Christmas with his dad and stepmom.

Upon our return from Alabama, Brian immediately went to his doctor who told him it was acid reflux and recommended Prilosec. He told Brian to call in two weeks if it wasn't helping. Brian never took the Prilosec because he knew that wasn't the problem, but he waited two weeks before going back. Again, I wish I would've pushed more.

When he went back to the doctor, they did an ultrasound of his gallbladder. That was fine, but they said, "There's a little something on your pancreas. It's subtle, but it's there." Yet, there was no sense of alarm or concern. They followed up with a CT scan two days later, which confirmed those findings. Still no sense of alarm or concern.

The day after the CT, Brian started feeling deep itching that could not be controlled. We thought he was having an allergic reaction to the dye they used for the scan. We called the doctor who said to take Benadryl and call back Monday if it persisted, which it did. It took over a week to get Brian scheduled for another test, during which time he itched so badly that he couldn't sleep. It was terrible.

It took three more tests, none of which were scheduled swiftly, before the cancer was diagnosed. Brian was a healthy thirty-eight year old who didn't smoke or drink, and lived a healthy lifestyle. There was apparently no reason to look for something like pancreatic cancer, so it took almost two months from his first appointment to the time he was diagnosed. In retrospect, they screwed up. As soon as they saw "a little something" on Brian's pancreas, and his tumor marker test came back elevated, they should have immediately referred him to a surgeon. If they had, Brian may still be here today.

*
KATHIE SCOTT
Kathie's 57-year-old husband Jim
died from prostate cancer in 2009

In our case, the pre-diagnosis symptom time period was relatively short. My husband was very good at ignoring symptoms and I didn't know he was having a problem until he told me his symptoms and said he needed to see a doctor. The appointment was made and, of course, I immediately took to the internet. I knew he was probably in trouble. It was as if my body and mind belonged to someone else, and I was floating above watching.

*
STEVE SHARP
Steve's 51-year-old wife Carolyn
died from melanoma in 2014

In November 2006, I noticed an eraser-size growth on Carolyn's right calf. She went to see her general practitioner in January 2007, who felt as though it was probably not significant. He biopsied it anyway just to be cautious. I'll never forget the look on Carolyn's face when she heard from the doctor that she had stage II melanoma. She had surgery to remove the cancer which was deemed a success. Her aftercare consisted of biannual total body exams by her dermatologist.

In July 2013, the cancer reappeared in her lymph nodes. In August 2013, it was discovered in her stomach. I'll forever wish I had pushed for yearly scans to make sure the cancer had not moved somewhere else in her body, unseen by her dermatologist.

*

DIANNE WEST
Dianne's husband Vern died from
multiple myeloma in 2010 at age 69

Vern was healthy and active. Although he had occasional back issues, he related that to playing a lot of sports in his younger years. Early in 2006, he started having severe back pain and did his usual routine of lying flat on a hard surface. When that didn't help, he visited a chiropractor. When those treatments didn't relieve the pain, the chiropractor recommended he see a medical doctor. We didn't suspect this was anything serious. Vern's job required a lot of running around the sports arena, up and down stairs, and standing on hard surfaces for long periods of time, so we assumed that had caused the issue.

Since he didn't see a doctor on a regular basis, he contacted the doctor who had handled his pancreatic cancer surgery some sixteen years previous. A CT scan didn't show anything, so the doctor referred Vern to a physical therapist. After one visit, his pain was much worse and he had difficulty walking. We contacted the doctor again and asked that he seek insurance approval for an MRI.

As soon as the MRI was done things moved very fast. Perhaps too fast. The doctor called the same day as the procedure to tell us there was a tumor on Vern's spine. He consulted a neuro and orthopedic surgeon and scheduled for us to meet the surgeon first thing the next morning. The surgeon wanted to perform the surgery the next day and sent us from his office to the hospital. We were in a state of shock. We never expected to hear the word cancer, but the urgency expressed by his doctor and the surgeon made us feel like we had to do whatever they recommended. On our way to the hospital, I asked Vern if we should get a second opinion, but he said no. He just wanted the tumor removed as quickly as possible.

Knowing how this all ended, I wish we had stopped to catch our breath and seek other opinions. But that would have taken time, and Vern was in severe pain and unable to walk. I've wondered whether any of his subsequent crises were caused by the wrong blood he received after this initial surgery. I do know that the abdominal aortic pseudoaneurysm that nearly killed him three years later was caused by a screw in the titanium cage they used to stabilize Vern's spine. He survived that surgery but went downhill quite severely afterward. It's easy to second-guess things after the fact, but I know we made the best decisions we could based on the information we had. There is no way to know how things might have turned out if we had done just one thing differently.

Vern had been diagnosed with pancreatic cancer in 1990, and scheduled for a Whipple procedure. During surgery, they found the tumor was benign. There was no medical explanation for it. We, and even his doctor, believed it was our miracle.

*

The greatest healing therapy
is friendship and love.

HUBERT H. HUMPHREY

*

SURVIVING LOSS BY CANCER

The greatest healing therapy
is friendship and love.

HUBERT H. HUMPHREY

*

CHAPTER THREE

Learning the Diagnosis

Start where you are. Use what you have.
Do what you can. ARTHUR ASHE

When a cancer diagnosis is delivered, our journeys often begin with shock and disbelief. From there, our emotions and reactions embark on a rollercoaster full of blinding twists and turns. How did your loved one handle the diagnosis? How well did you understand the prognosis?

*

JANICE DEL VECCHIO
Janice lost her husband Stephen to bile duct cancer in 2006 at age 47,
and her second husband John to pancreatic cancer in 2013 at age 55

Steve initially handled the news of his illness pretty well and was positive that maybe some kind of treatment would work and he would be cured. That was short lived and reality started to set in for both of us. I was in shock mode but immediately went into warp mode, and was determined to find the best treatment available. I would use my connections at work to find the best doctor and treatment. I got him an appointment at Beth Israel in Boston with the top oncologist for this type of cancer. We felt some relief after the initial consultation, and additional tests and scans were ordered. The oncologist said he couldn't confirm the type of cancer Steve had, as the quality of testing by the original hospital was very poor. That gave us a shred of hope that maybe we would get lucky and it would be a treatable cancer. The hardest part for both of us was waiting for the test results. The doctor said that waiting was the hardest part. It truly was.

Beth Israel confirmed the diagnosis and Steve began treatment. Admittedly, once I knew the final results, there was a sense of relief in not having to angst over the test results any longer. Now that we knew what type of cancer he had, we could make a plan. What brought us hope was going from no treatment options to having options. We also believed in the power of prayer, which brought tremendous comfort.

John and I were both devastated by the news. We knew that pancreatic cancer was a deadly disease without many options. Again, I went into warp mode and got John an appointment with the top pancreatic oncologist at Massachusetts General Hospital in Boston. Similar to my experience with my first husband, MGH wanted to do their own testing. Testing was repeated but were inconclusive, which caused more tests and more waiting.

Ultimately, a biopsy was done. We met with the oncologist and radiologist who said the biopsy showed pancreatic cancer. We both looked at each other with our jaws dropped. Blood tests and additional scans confirmed the original diagnosis.

I had more of an understanding of the diagnosis than John did, as I had been down this route before. John was an extremely optimistic person and was hopeful that he would have success with his treatment. That helped me tremendously. Again, the results were back, we knew what we were up against and a plan was formulated. I became John's healthcare advocate and cheerleader, as well as being his wife, who was scared to death of the outcome.

*

CYNTHIA HORACEK
Cynthia's husband Don died from
rectal cancer in 2010 at age 57

Don handled the diagnosis very well with a positive attitude. I cried and told him he wasn't allowed to die.

*

MARGARET HUTSELL
Margaret's 77-year-old husband Tom
died from pancreatic cancer in 2016

Our world collapsed with a simple phone call from a physician we had never met while in the car on our way home from the grocery store. The bluetooth phone connection was still new to us so when the phone rang, we pushed a few buttons and answered. A voice asked if this was Tom he was talking with. When Tom said it was, the voice explained that the CT results were back, and without skipping a beat, had revealed a pancreatic mass. Dr. L wanted to see us the following Monday morning and would work us into his schedule. That was it! This was a colleague of our doctor whom we had never met or spoken with. He told us the results and hung up. Tom's first words were "Dead man walking," and I began to cry, what was to become a routine behavior. We had no idea what lay ahead nor how bad it would be, and wouldn't find out for another week.

We met with the oncologist the following Thursday afternoon, and the diagnosis of pancreatic cancer stage II was made. The tumor was 1.3 cm and there was no apparent spread of additional tumors seen on the CT. Chemotherapy would be started and we were going to beat this thing since Tom was one of the lucky ones to have it diagnosed at an early stage. Whipple surgery down the road would most likely give us a reasonable chance for a cure. We were scared to death and yet thrilled to have a hopeful outcome.

Chemo was started, weight loss began, and eating became a chore. Tom's bilirubin was excessively elevated and until it got down to a normal range, no surgery would be scheduled. So began the routine of chemo, alternated with hydrating fluids and pills hoping to stop the weight loss due to the poor appetite Tom was now experiencing and issues with his digestive juices enabling him to get nutritional elements into his body on a daily basis. Thousands of dollars (yep, you are reading this right) were spent on capsules that were supposed to help with digestion but, in reality, had to be taken with so much water before each meal or snack, Tom was no longer hungry after taking them. This nutritional merry-go-round lasted for two months when our oncologist finally suggested that since Tom still had his pancreas he did not need the meds.

We were going through the motions of normalcy and the only times we were even halfway comfortable with anything that was going on was when we were at home, with our wee dog, simply doing the stuff we had always done.

*

LYNN JORDAAN
Lynn's 58-year-old husband Johan
died from esophageal cancer in 2014

He was very philosophical once the diagnosis came in. Being a left brain analytical engineer, he hopped onto the internet to find all these cures everyone was saying were miracles. He had decided very early on that there would be no chemotherapy, radiation, nor surgery. I, on the other hand, was all gung-ho for exactly the things he was against. I mean, those were conventional treatment, were they not?

It was quickly pointed out that the cancer was terminal, especially since he did not want conventional treatment. No one could give us a timeline exactly, but he was told to get his affairs in order.

The one thing that brought comfort was that we still had one another for whatever time was left. I chose to honor his wishes, and supported the unconventional vitamin B_{12}, vitamin C infusions, etc.

He decided he wasn't feeling any better and consented to visit an oncologist, who promptly sat him down and told him she could offer chemo and radiation. He chose the chemo which worked quite well at first, but he was fighting a losing battle.

*

GAIL MARCHESA
Gail's husband John died from
colon cancer in 2009 at age 55

Upon first learning the diagnosis, it was like, "Okay, now what?" But still thinking "Oh, it'll be fine." As time goes on, that's not the case. I learned a lot, and got mad a lot. John, at that point, accepted it and went with the flow.

*

HEATHER MCLAUGHLIN
Heather's 35-year-old husband Derek
died from colorectal cancer in 2013

We didn't handle the news well. We initially thought they were lying, but knew something was wrong. We saw specialists who told us the same thing, colon cancer, stage IIIB. We didn't have time to think. Honestly, we barely had time to breathe, and we really didn't understand the prognosis.

Derek and I wanted children but no one made sure we understood the risks of radiation, and that he likely would be sterile. I remember a whirlwind of people telling us what to do, where to go, and how to act. We just made the movements. I don't know if we really had time to sit down and talk with each other, cry with each other. I wish we would have had that.

*

SUE NOVA
Sue's husband Dana died from
lung cancer in 2012 at age 46

After we got to Chicago, Dana immediately made an appointment with a pulmonologist. She went over his results, did tests of her own, and told him we needed to contact a thoracic surgeon to determine the next course of action, which was surgical. The opinion was that if this was cancer, surgical removal would be best. Keep in mind, at this point we had no idea whether this was cancer or something else.

A minimally invasive wedge resection was scheduled. They planned to go between Dana's ribs to remove the affected lung section, send the spot to pathology to determine whether it was cancer, and then proceed accordingly. I was asleep in the waiting room when the surgeon came in, woke me, and said it was cancer localized to that spot. They successfully removed it and were closing Dana up. I don't remember what I felt. Cancer . . . removed it all . . . successful surgery.

When I saw Dana in recovery, I realized he had no idea what had happened, what the outcome was or anything. As he began to come out of the anesthesia, in between screams of pain and morphine, he asked what happened. I probably told him ten times what the results were. We now assumed he was cancer free. How wrong we were.

We returned to California in 2010. Dana continued to see an oncologist for routine CT scans. Things went well for months. Until we got the call to come in and see the doctor. We got to the cancer center and went back into one of the rooms. Dana's regular doctor wasn't in yet, but one of the visiting physicians was. We chatted a little bit and she blurted out something about the cancer. Apparently the look on our faces let her know we had no idea what she was talking about. She apologized profusely and quickly stepped out of the room.

Dana's regular doctor came in a few minutes later and told us a couple spots had appeared on Dana's lung and had grown since the last CT scan. A course of chemo and radiation would begin soon. We knew well enough that the survival rate for lung cancer wasn't good. What followed was a two-year fight literally to the death.

*

SHERYL POCHEL
Sheryl's husband Brian died from
pancreatic cancer in 2011 at age 43

Prior to his diagnosis, Brian researched pancreas cancer online. I wasn't home when he got the phone call that told him this could be a possibility.

"There is some concern of a tumor, but I still think we are dealing with Pancreatitis," the doctor said.

All Brian needed to hear was pancreas and tumor and he was off doing research. I got home and he was sitting on the bed crying. He told me they thought it was cancer with a twenty-five percent survival rate the first year.

I misunderstood and said, "Well, that means seventy-five percent live, right? That isn't so bad."

He corrected me. "No. Seventy-five percent die within their first year."

Numb. I went numb. That night, as we laid in bed, neither of us slept. We just laid there holding hands all night long.

I was thirty-six, Brian was thirty-eight, and we had four young kids ages six, four, two and ten months. We were self-employed, he as a chiropractor and I ran his clinic. Neither one of us could comprehend what was happening. Neither of us could see him dying from this.

Once he was officially diagnosed, Brian asked his oncologist how long he had. The response was, "Well, so, a year, probably not two."

At that time Brian was diagnosed as having stage IIIB pancreatic adenocarcinoma. The IIIB meant they could see no spread of disease, but were unable to remove it because of its location and proximity to major veins and arteries. We were lucky in that Brian survived for five and a half years. We rarely talked about his cancer being terminal because he always rallied from every complication, and there were many. It wasn't until January 2011, when we started to see the end.

*

KATHIE SCOTT
Kathie's 57-year-old husband Jim
died from prostate cancer in 2009

He was understandably upset and worried when the news was delivered. The oncologist that he eventually chose to treat him did not mince any words as to the seriousness of the situation. He made sure we understand that this condition could not be cured, but could be managed for several years. He said if we had things to do and places to go, we should take care of it. There was no mistaking the prognosis.

*

STEVE SHARP
Steve's 51-year-old wife Carolyn
died from melanoma in 2014

Carolyn had surgery to remove the cancerous lymph nodes and was able to take medication that eradicated the cancer in her stomach, and we were elated. But in May 2014, cancer was found in her brain.

When told that time was short and she had probably four months to live, we were in shock. We both understood the seriousness of the situation but received conflicting news. Carolyn's oncologist believed she had more time—perhaps two more years. We found comfort and hope by electing to believe the oncologist's viewpoint, and were optimistic that if ninety-five percent of patients died with a terminal diagnosis, my wife would be among the five percent who beat it.

Carolyn was a tremendous fighter and we believed she was going to make it. Finally, both the neurologist and oncologist said she had only two weeks to live, and we realized her situation was terminal. During this difficult time, I was comforted by my faith and from the tremendous support of family and friends.

*

AUDRA THEROUX
Audra's father died from
esophageal cancer in 2014

My father handled his diagnosis like a pro, like the Marine that he was. This is his exact quote from his Facebook page about his diagnosis:

"Well today I start another mission in life! I was diagnosed with cancer yesterday and am now making arrangements to start and kick its ass! I'm not a quitter and will fight hard to achieve my goal! I have a lot of support to win my battle!"

The biopsy results came in right before I was due to fly home from vacation. When I talked to my father about it, this is what he told me, word for word. I never forgot. I never will.

"Lots of things in life have tried to kill me. I've been to war and back and survived. Cancer will not kill me. I'm tough!"

So, I would say he handled it just like he would any challenge, head on and ready to fight.

My dad was the type of person to go with the flow and take things as they happened. Me? I like to research everything and learn about what is happening. If I am going to take a new medication, I want to know what it is and how it works. So, with my father's diagnosis, I set to work researching not only esophageal cancer, but also cancer in general. I wanted to know how I could help my father, make him more comfortable, and most importantly, what he could eat.

With the tumor in his esophagus, it was hard for him to eat. So I did a lot of research on foods that he was able to eat, and set to work making those for him. My dad loved food—mostly sweets. Losing his ability to eat was probably one of the hardest things for him. So I was always trying to find things that he was able to eat.

If I'm honest, as someone who researches everything, I never researched the prognosis on esophageal cancer. I know I did this on purpose. I don't think I really wanted to know. I didn't want to read something horrible (and trust me, esophageal cancer IS horrible and is a very fast death and almost always terminal). I felt like if I read bad news, that it would affect the way I treated him, and in turn, it would affect his fighting spirit, and that was the last thing I wanted. So, I avoided the prognosis all together. I didn't research it, and we never discussed it with the doctor. We always focused on his treatment and what we could do to help him. Interestingly, the doctor never actually brought it up either.

After I lost my father, the doctor told me that I never asked about it, so it was never discussed. My dad was not one to ask questions. That was part of the reason why I went to all his doctor appointments and chemo sessions, notebook in hand, making sure I had all the available information. There was so much new information being presented, I knew I couldn't just absorb it all at the appointments, so I wrote it down to go back to at a later date. Plus, my dad's sister is a nurse. I always discussed his appointments with her over the phone, since she lived in South Carolina.

This may sound ridiculous given the fact that my dad had cancer, but the thought never actually passed through my mind that he might die. My dad was the toughest man I knew. When he told me he was going to beat cancer, I believed that. Maybe it was because I needed to believe it, but I really, truly believed it in my heart. Even when he got worse, I still thought he would get through it. I know lots of people get sick during treatment, but they still come through the other side. I thought for sure that would be my dad.

I didn't realize his cancer was terminal until he was in the hospital and had a PET scan which revealed disturbing results. The doctor called me that night to go over the results, and then asked to meet with me and my mother the next day.

My dad's doctor was the head of oncology. When we met with him the next day, he said the cancer was terminal and Dad had about six months to live. He wanted to get Dad set up for palliative care and hospice so that they could keep him comfortable. To say that was a shock would be an understatement. I was at every single appointment with Dad. Nothing had suggested to me that he was going to die. I was in utter shock. I don't remember the rest of the meeting. We met with the palliative care nurse and a social worker, and Dad was discharged that day. The hospice nurse would meet with us the next morning to get him set up in the program.

I spent that night in shock. I can't remember it. Dad didn't seem shocked at all. After he died, we learned that he suspected he was going to die. Like I mentioned, he just wasn't one to complain.

The next morning was Saturday, and the hospice nurse came. I really believe hospice nurses are angels on earth. They are wonderful. My father was in so much pain, she wanted to admit him to the facility for a few days to get his pain under control and get the things she needed for home care. It was no easy feat but we managed to talk my father into going. On Saturday afternoon, he walked into the hospice building. He refused a wheelchair—he walked into the building.

On Sunday morning, he passed away. On Friday afternoon I learned that Dad's cancer was terminal, and he died Sunday morning at 10:25 a.m. I don't think I had time to fully comprehend what was happening or to make peace with the situation. It all happened so fast.

*

DIANNE WEST
Dianne's husband Vern died from
multiple myeloma in 2010 at age 69

Vern was not one to openly share his feelings. When his best friend died during our first year of marriage, he was devastated but wouldn't talk about it. It drove me nuts, because I need to talk to think. He did not. So he allowed me to talk and I allowed him to be silent. And that worked well for us during our forty-one years together.

When we first heard the diagnosis, he reacted as expected. I knew he was scared but I also knew I could not push him to talk about it because that would not be helpful for him. I gave him a few minutes to process it after the doctor left the room. He asked if he was going to die. And I told him no, that we were going to fight this with everything we had and we would win. I believed that with my whole heart. And Vern did believe he would beat this cancer. Throughout each crises, he never lost hope. Oh, there were times he hit bottom, but he allowed me to pull him back up. I worked hard to keep him positive because I believed that would make a difference.

I didn't see it while we were living it, but I can now look back through my journal and see a turning point about three months before he died. He was so tired of everything and was ready for it to end. I was not. I had never heard of multiple myeloma, so I spent a lot of time researching and joining online groups of myeloma patients and their caregivers to share information and ask questions. Vern was happy letting me handle all of that and didn't want to know much of the details. I used the information I gathered to be able to ask the right questions when we'd meet with his oncologist.

I knew from my research that myeloma is not curable, but it can be treatable for some, so that was my focus. He had so many medical crises but each time I believed he would survive. That was the only way I knew how to do this hard work. I really didn't accept that he was actually going to die until we made the decision to move into hospice.

Friends who suddenly lose a loved one often assume we talked about his death during those cancer years and settled all sorts of things that they didn't have the opportunity to, but that was just not the case for us. We never spoke about him dying until those final four days of his life when he was in hospice. And at that point, he did not speak much at all.

A hero is an ordinary individual who finds the
strength to persevere and endure in spite of
overwhelming obstacles.

CHRISTOPHER REEVE
*

A hero is an ordinary individual who finds the
strength to persevere and endure in spite of
overwhelming obstacles.

CHAPTER FOUR

Telling Others

Sometimes the transition from being in control
of your life to having absolutely no control is swift,
but other times it is so gradual that you wonder
exactly when it truly began. -MICKEY ROONEY

As we begin our journey through cancer, so too must our family and friends. For some, facing the challenges together can strengthen family bonds. For others, the stress may create new or worsening problems. When did you tell family members about the cancer diagnosis? How did they react?

*

JANICE DEL VECCHIO
Janice lost her husband Stephen to bile duct cancer in 2006 at age 47,
and her second husband John to pancreatic cancer in 2013 at age 55

Steve's family did not react well to the news. His parents were divorced and they had no relationship with each other at all. Steve had a relationship with his dad but they were not very close. He had a sister and they were not close to her either. Steve's mom was a very nice and sweet person. She was understandably upset and just couldn't seem to fathom that her son was seriously ill and likely would pass away at some point. He kept his family on a need to know basis, and felt that was best. He knew his mother was not going to be able to cope with what was happening, which was very hard on him. I told him that she, of course, was going to be upset and may never fully grasp what's going on, but that she was his mom and he should make an effort to be as compassionate as he could.

As a couple, we decided we didn't want to know how long Steve had left. His doctor too felt it wasn't in his patient's best interest to have an estimate of time left, otherwise folks seemed to focus on what they are told about life expectancy versus enjoying each day.

My family was the most supportive of all. Steve and I spent a lot of years with my family and he was fairly close with everyone. My sisters and their husbands took him to appointments from time to time to give me break and visited with him on a regular basis. His family never offered to take him to treatment or help us in any way. We were actually glad they didn't, as Steve didn't want to deal with family drama. It wasn't until the end of his life that his sister, her husband, and his father tried to intervene and interfere with decisions being made in regard to his care and final funeral arrangements. It really added a tremendous amount of stress to an already stressful situation. I had to get the hospital, hospice, and our priest involved to end the interfering. Of course, I was always getting the brunt of their aggression but I brushed it off and did what I had to do.

John's family did not take the news about John's illness well at all. They were very upset about it, understandably so, as John's mother was very ill and actively dying at the time. John didn't want her to know. She constantly asked me what was going on with John and I just told her repeatedly that he was having some stomach issues. John and I also didn't want the doctor to tell us how long he could expect to live. His doctor shared the same philosophy as my first husband's doctor did. His brothers and sisters wanted to know how long and we told them we didn't know, so please drop it.

John had two children, a daughter and son. His daughter lived around the corner from us while his son lived out of state. I can only imagine how heartbreaking the news about their father was to them, as their mother took her own life a few years earlier. I tried to keep them updated on what was happening. John's son was appreciative and came home to see his dad as often as he could.

John's daughter asked me to not call her and give her any details about her dad. She preferred I tell her husband who would relay the information. She rarely visited her dad while he was ill, never offered to make any meals, clean the house or bring her son over to see his grandfather. This was heartbreaking to her dad, but she never knew about it, as I never said anything to her about it. I felt it was not my place to do so.

John called me one day while I was at work to tell me he had a temperature of 104.1 and the hospital wanted him to come into the emergency room. It didn't make sense for me to come home to drive him in due to the urgency of the situation. I said I would ask my sister or her husband to drive him in and I would meet them at the hospital, but John wanted his daughter to give him a ride. Sadly, she refused to do it. John's neighbor offered to babysit her son, but she still wouldn't do it. Ultimately, his neighbor drove John to the emergency room and I met them there. John nearly fell out of the car once he got there. I was very angry about her not helping her dad but as time passed, I realized that she just couldn't do it for some reason, and would have to deal with the consequence of her decision.

John's mom died four months before John. This was tough, but also a relief as she was very ill and John no longer had to worry about her finding out about his diagnosis. John's son quit his job, moved home, and lived with me for two weeks when we found out that his dad was actively dying. What an amazing kid, and what joy and peace he brought to his dad when he needed him. My family was also there for me. They were very supportive, and are to this day.

*

CYNTHIA HORACEK
Cynthia's husband Don died from
rectal cancer in 2010 at age 57

It's so hard to say how they reacted to the news. Don didn't want to tell our daughters because he didn't want them to worry, but we discussed it and he realized they needed to know because if he died, it would be too much of a shock. They seemed to handle it well; there were no dramatics.

Don wouldn't tell his father, though. He said if his dad heard the C word, he would just worry. My parents knew, and I can't remember much of what was said but my father was a physician and he took it pretty stoically. Don's brother acknowledged the news, but they didn't really show emotions, so he was pretty much blasé about it.

*

MARGARET HUTSELL
Margaret's 77-year-old husband Tom
died from pancreatic cancer in 2016

Our kids were terrified. Their spouses were terrified. Our grand-children, who are mostly adults at this point, were terrified. Losing this husband, father, grandfather, mentor, and counsel for us all, who was an articulate and loving man was beyond comprehension.

Our son in Illinois started visiting once a month and phoned his dad daily. The two local kids spent weekends here and invited us both to spend hours of just being together when Tom felt good enough to leave our home. We felt love coming from friends we had not seen in years. Through posts on Caringbridge.org, we reconnected with folks from all over the world who we had once been either in business with, volunteered together, or shared the child raising days way back when.

Tom and I decided our bucket list was to continue to "keep on keeping on" and we wanted to do it right here in our home, trying to be what we were as long as we possibly could. The two of us spent hours talking about what might lie ahead and what we would do. Our feelings were on the table from day one. We cried together, held each other, smiled as often as we could, and just lived our lives. We did just what we wanted to do with only those we wanted to do it with, and focused on comfort and hope for more time. There would never be enough time.

*

LYNN JORDAAN
Lynn's 58-year-old husband Johan
died from esophageal cancer in 2014

He chose to email updates of every procedure to our family and friends, mainly to keep his sister from flying from Zimbabwe to nurse him. We were as open to everyone as we could be. The only one we sort of kept things from was our daughter, who was planning a wedding at the time. We didn't want her to move up the wedding date. We did, however, keep her fiancé completely in the loop, and charged him with divulging information as required. There was a mixture of keeping up a strong front and honest emotion going on, depending on who we were dealing with at the time. Between us, we expressed emotions as freely and raw as humanly possible. There were many tears, much laughter, and a lot of rambling down memory lane.

*

GAIL MARCHESA
Gail's husband John died from
colon cancer in 2009 at age 55

Shocked is the only word for it. Some were just stupid and I wanted to slap them silly. Everybody had an opinion of what to do, ugh! Other than that, okay.

72

*

HEATHER MCLAUGHLIN
Heather's 35-year-old husband Derek
died from colorectal cancer in 2013

The family was shocked. One thing that Derek was good at was making jokes and making light of a situation. He had colorectal cancer. He called it butt cancer. It's what I still call it today. He used to say, "Why can't I get a cool cancer like brain cancer? I had to get butt cancer..." I am sorry for those who lost a loved one to brain cancer. Derek smiled and laughed and in turn it made the people around him do the same, but he was so very sick. It took people a long time to realize that, because he didn't look that way.

*

SUE NOVA
Sue's husband Dana died from
lung cancer in 2012 at age 46

We were all elated that surgery had successfully removed the spots. We were open regarding his treatment. We had no reason to believe he was going to die. He was feeling good, aside from the down days with chemo. He was working, traveling . . . we were living. Until May 2012, we held out hope.

*

SHERYL POCHEL
Sheryl's husband Brian died from
pancreatic cancer in 2011 at age 43

Our immediate family was stunned. Many of them were at the hospital with us when Brian was officially diagnosed. In the days and weeks that followed, they helped us immensely. Some did research to find what was working as far as cancer treatments, others helped with the kids. My brother looked into different financial things for me. Overall though, everyone was extremely sad. Sad for Brian, sad for me, sad for our children. No one could see me without him, as we had been together since high school. It was a very difficult time for everyone.

The hardest part was telling our two oldest girls, who were four and six. My oldest daughter's birthday is in February, and even now she equates it with her dad being diagnosed with cancer. They were young. They didn't understand and it was hard to grasp how they would manage this at such a young age. My heart still hurts for my children. They didn't get a chance to really truly know who their dad was and what an incredible person he could be.

*

KATHIE SCOTT
Kathie's 57-year-old husband Jim
died from prostate cancer in 2009

Three daughters being told their dad was very sick and going to require a lot of treatment wasn't easy. Nobody wants to hear that some one you dearly love has cancer. We did not tell them exactly what the doctor said, but it soon became clear to them how it was going to be. They were obviously devastated and in shock.

His siblings had always looked to him for support and answers and it rocked their world, to say the least. We kept up the strong face and positive attitude to the end.

Only one of our three daughters could talk to me and ask the hard questions. Maybe, being the oldest, she was elected but I don't know for sure. I kept my dark thoughts and emotions completely inside the entire time. I had a couple of close friends who I could open up to in the darkest times, and for that I will be eternally grateful.

*

STEVE SHARP
Steve's 51-year-old wife Carolyn
died from melanoma in 2014

The entire family was shocked when we learned the diagnosis was terminal. We truly thought we had more time together. Carolyn's mother immediately came down from Connecticut to stay with us. All of us finally understood the prognosis was terminal, and handled it as best we could.

Our youngest child was finishing her senior year of high school, and had a terrible time dealing with all the questions and well-wishes since her mother had taught there. Carolyn's father was dealing with the horror of seeing both Carolyn and his wife, Carolyn's stepmother, struggle with terminal cancer.

During Carolyn's final days, we made the most of our time. We watched our youngest child graduate, buried my father at Arlington National Cemetery, sent our daughter off to college, and made one last trip to the beach. Looking back, I wish our family had talked more about Carolyn's pending death, and that she had been able to leave letters and videos for her loved ones to have in the coming years.

*

AUDRA THEROUX
Audra's father died from
esophageal cancer in 2014

When we got the news about my father, I think most of us were shocked. In my thirty-nine years of life to that point, I had never seen my father complain about anything. He was basically a rock. He was my rock. I think it hit most of us the same way—we couldn't believe it was happening. My father, though, was so solid with the news. The absolute conviction that he would beat it, I think, helped all of us. We were supportive and tried to treat him the same way we always had (because that was the only thing he would accept from us).

I was my dad's cancer buddy, meaning that I went to all of my dad's appointments. Where he went, I went. I became the one who passed along Dad's health information, including to his sister in South Carolina. I became the go-to for those who wanted accurate and complete information.

If you were to ever ask my dad how his appointment went, he'd answer "fine," or "I still have cancer." Always a joker. I don't know if he wasn't taking everything in (granted, it was a lot of information all thrown at you at one time), or if he just wasn't listening. You could never count on him for any real information about his health, though, so my family came to me. I had a lot of talks with my aunt (my dad's sister) about everything, and my notebooks full of information from the appointments came in handy. There was absolutely no way to remember everything that the doctors and nurses told us, not to mention that there were lots of strange new words to learn. My aunt was a nurse by profession, so I tried to give her as much information as I could, so she was fully updated on how my dad was doing. Giving her all the information was also helpful to me. Since she was a medical professional, she could explain what some of the information meant, or test results, without me having to look it up.

I was always honest and forthcoming with everyone about how my dad was doing. I kept track of his weight, what he ate, lab results, what the doctors said, etc. Basically, I felt responsible for him and his cancer. That probably sounds strange and totally unreasonable, but that was how I felt.

When we got news on Friday afternoon that my father had only six months to live, that was the first time I did not immediately call my aunt to share the news. I just couldn't do it. The next morning when hospice came and got Dad admitted to the facility, we obviously had to call and let her know. But I still couldn't talk to her. I was having feelings of extreme guilt, like I had somehow failed my father, and failed to make him healthy. I didn't know how to tell her that her only brother was going to die. In the past year and a half, my aunt had lost both parents, and now she was going to lose her brother, too. I was still reeling with the news that my father was going to die, I was blaming myself, and I couldn't find the strength to tell her. My mother called to tell her because I couldn't do it. That was the only time I was unable to communicate with my family about my father. I was too wrapped up in my own pain and guilt at that time.

*

DIANNE WEST
Dianne's husband Vern died from
multiple myeloma in 2010 at age 69

Vern's parents and only sibling all died before his diagnosis. My parents were both gone, and my siblings all lived over two thousand miles away. They expressed concern but none came out during the four years we dealt with cancer, nor did they come for Vern's service or in the years following his death. I had real anger about that for longer than I should have, but finally realized that it is what it is, and holding onto anger was only hurting me. I forgave them though admit that I have not forgotten.

Our adult son was going through personal issues at the time, so I did protect him from the really hard stuff. He is much like his father about not showing his feelings.

I wrote extensively about what we were going through in my Caring Bridge journal, but didn't share my true emotions. I suppose I expected those who were reading my posts to know I wasn't sharing everything, that they would recognize how horrible things were at times and just show up. That only happened a couple of times during those four long years.

I wish I could have asked for what I needed, but I could not. I did ask for what Vern needed, for people to visit or call him, but that didn't happen often either. It was disappointing, but I really didn't have the time to think about it that much. Another time for my "it is what it is" phrase.

The act of writing each day was quite therapeutic for me, a good release. And I've appreciated having that journal to refer to even now. Using Caring Bridge as my means of communication allowed me to put our story out there for those who were interested. It was so much easier than having to maintain a massive email distribution list; caringbridge.org/visit/vernwest/journal.

*

Anything is possible when you have the right
people there to support you.

MISTY COPELAND
*

CHAPTER FIVE

The Physical Changes

The bereaved need more than just the space
to grieve the loss. They also need the space to
grieve the transition. -LYNDA CHELDELIN FELL

Cancer and its treatment are hard on the body, resulting in physical changes that are sometimes unexpected. While some are short-term, like baldness, others are permanent. For loved ones, these changes can be shocking. How prepared were you for the physical changes caused by cancer and its treatment?

*

JANICE DEL VECCHIO
Janice lost her husband Stephen to bile duct cancer in 2006 at age 47,
and her second husband John to pancreatic cancer in 2013 at age 55

I was not prepared at all, especially with my first husband. It's so heartbreaking to watch someone you love slowly deteriorate. The changes are subtle in the beginning. As the illness goes on, it's hard seeing them become so exhausted from treatment. I dreaded the day before treatments, hoping bloods tests indicated it was safe for them to have treatment, seeing the disappointment and anguish on their faces when the doctor determines it's not safe for them to have chemo that day. It is devastating to watch. I was scared for myself, but felt I needed to hide it for the sake of my husbands. It's hard being the sole support system, but I did my best.

The decrease in social activities was very hard. We had to miss several weddings, parties, and various other social events as both were too sick to attend. It wasn't about my feelings, but theirs. They wanted desperately to go, and it was hard to watch their disappointment. They both would apologize profusely. I did my best to reassure both that it was okay, and that maybe later on when they felt better, we could attend activities and invite friends and family over.

I was better prepared for when my second husband became ill. I knew from experience what to expect, but it didn't make it any easier to accept. The absolute scariest change in both husbands was the loss of their sense of humor. Both loved to joke and laugh, and when that was gone, I knew it was getting close to the end.

*

CYNTHIA HORACEK
Cynthia's husband Don died from
rectal cancer in 2010 at age 57

Because Don had Crohn's disease, a chronic illness, the physical changes were not all that shocking. He was down to one hundred ten pounds when he had surgery to remove the tumor, but he was always underweight. That's about the only physical change he underwent.

I did begin to notice he had chemo brain after a few months. His driving became less safe and I told him he had to stop driving. He seemed to handle that well. After his death, I went to balance the checkbook and noticed it hadn't been balanced in a while—something he always did because he was a CPA. That shocked me.

In the final month, Don got weaker and weaker and began to use a walker around the house. When we got home from a hospital stay or doctor's appointment, he could barely make it into the bedroom, even with help. It was hard to watch. That was very scary for me. I was always afraid he'd pass out in the hallway and I wouldn't be able to get him to the bed. I would encourage him and tell him to just hold on, just a little bit further. Somehow, he managed to make it.

The very end was hardest, of course, because he began to bleed out. His nose bled, his gums bled, and I know he was having brain bleeds because he wasn't lucid much during the final few days.

*

MARGARET HUTSELL
Margaret's 77-year-old husband Tom
died from pancreatic cancer in 2016

Tom's eyes and skin began to show signs of jaundice about the time the itching began. We thought it would resolve once the elevated bilirubin levels started to decline. That didn't happen and Tom needed to have a biliary catheter inserted soon after diagnosis. This procedure was so stressful. Finding out that Tom also needed to attach a bag for the bile to drain into, which needed to be drained twice a day, was nerve-wracking. Little did I know that this was just the beginning.

The weight loss and inability to eat what Tom had always eaten became apparent soon after. He had always been a robust man and active daily. His passion for gardening and working in our yard was now tempered by chemo infusions and trying to be comfortable with this new thing hanging out of his right side. We were happy there was no nausea or vomiting after chemo treatments, but Tom developed a sensitivity to cold. Even in the heat of the summer and fall months, Tom wore his "uniform" of sweats and even a jacket.

*

LYNN JORDAAN
Lynn's 58-year-old husband Johan
died from esophageal cancer in 2014

I think I sort of knew what to expect. Johan did not have a lot of hair loss, but the scariest thing was that he did lose an awful amount of weight. He started the journey at two hundred and seventy pounds, and weighed ninety-eight pounds when he died. It felt like he was just slowly withering away and that at any moment he would float away in the ether, which I suppose is exactly what he did in the end.

He was pretty stable as far as emotions were concerned, up until a few weeks before he died. He became agitated and irritable and said he was running out of time, that he still hadn't taught my daughter and I all he thought we ought to know. He was exhausted and couldn't concentrate, and was starting to leave his copious emails to friends and family to me. He half dictated, half told me what it was he needed said, leaving me to put it into words. This must have been difficult, as he was always editing anything I wrote!

The scariest thing, I think, was watching this man who was so big in both stature and presence fade away. I still look at pictures and feel shaken at how drawn and thin he was at the end of his life.

*

GAIL MARCHESA
Gail's husband John died from
colon cancer in 2009 at age 55

John lost weight but mainly looked the same. He was more willing to accept help and it was in the last two weeks that the physical changes came. One time, I had thought that he banged up his legs because they were bruised, but the hospice nurse said it happens when the organs are shutting down. I had a lot of cold chills run through me because of the change. I will never forget the way he looked!

*

HEATHER MCLAUGHLIN
Heather's 35-year-old husband Derek
died from colorectal cancer in 2013

I thought I was prepared. In the beginning, Derek really didn't change much. It wasn't until after the big surgery at the Cleveland clinic in Florida when he really changed. Physically, he lost so much weight. He got to be just about my size, or a little larger. He started losing his hair but in true Derek fashion, he beat the drugs to it and just shaved it all off. He didn't want clumps of it falling out.

Once all this happened, it really took a toll on me. My husband didn't look like my husband any more. It was so hard to look at him with a permanent bladder bag, a permanent colostomy, sunken face, no hair, and just no hope. At this point, his mind was starting to slip. Derek was normally very sharp, so this was difficult to watch and deal with—taking away his car keys, repeating myself over and over, asking him over and over what he wanted to eat.

The hardest part was when we lost hope. We had reached a point when all the news became bad news. It got harder and harder. Harder than I ever thought. Seeing his body deteriorate was very hard. When his organs started to shut down, his legs turned a horrible blackish-blue color and the rest of his body was yellow from jaundice. But in the end, when he was able to talk to me, he was still the same sweet Derek. I do everything in my power to remember those moments and not the visual image of his body at the end.

*

SUE NOVA
Sue's husband Dana died from
lung cancer in 2012 at age 46

Obviously, we anticipated hair loss. Since my husband already shaved his head, that wasn't really an issue. One thing that did happen was that the remaining hair on his body thinned considerably. He was Italian and Greek, so he was quite fuzzy.

During his clinical trial, the drug he was taking caused him to break out in pimples and pustules on his face, on his head, and also on his back. Through it all he continued working and carrying on as if his skin was completely normal. I admired him so much for being that way. I am not sure I could have been so confident!

The weight loss, the weakness, and how confused and completely incapacitated he was were also hard. Once, I had to go to the pharmacy to pick up his meds. I told him to stay in bed and I would be back in five minutes. Well, when I got home a, there he was on the ground along with his walker halfway out the front door. I got him up and onto the couch, and then asked what happened. He said that after I left, someone rang the doorbell but by the time he got there they were gone. He was so apologetic and looked so defeated that it just killed me. I'm pretty sure that was the last time I ever left him unattended.

*

SHERYL POCHEL
Sheryl's husband Brian died from
pancreatic cancer in 2011 at age 43

Before Brian was diagnosed, his only issue was being overweight. He was five-foot-eight and weighed two hundred forty pounds at his heaviest. As his cancer progressed, even before he was diagnosed, he started losing weight, sometimes a pound a day. It was scary. His low weight through cancer was one hundred eighty-five pounds, which seemed much too skinny for him. He was able to level off around one hundred ninety pounds, which actually looked good on him.

Once Brian started chemo, at the very first sign of hair loss, he chose to shave his head. My teasing words of, "I hope you never go bald because you have a big head," spoken long before cancer had come back to haunt me. However, much to my surprise, Brian was an extremely handsome bald man. He had a perfectly shaped head, and I know this to be true, because I had several women comment on how hot he looked! It was funny, and made him feel a little better about it. The ironic thing is that Brian always needed to shave his head to stay bald. I told him at one point that he should just let it grow and see what happened, but he refused to do that until the very end of his treatment. Once he did, his hair came back just fine and he said, "Why have I been shaving this whole time?" All I could do was shake my head.

Over the course of five and a half years, Brian had many surgeries. The first was eight months after his diagnosis. The surgeon said we should attempt the Whipple surgery. They removed his gallbladder, bile duct, part of his stomach, part of his small intestine and a third of his pancreas. It was a massive surgery that left a huge scar across his abdomen, and dealing with his pain was hard.

Fifteen months later he was diagnosed with a brain tumor, which they removed. They shaved his hair in that area and when they stitched him up he looked like a baseball. Our daughter was eight at the time and terrified of him. She wouldn't go near him for a while. There were other surgeries too, radiation burns, a lot of fatigue that kept Brian from enjoying family time, but none of it compared to the changes that happened in 2011.

One night in January 2011, I went to give Brian a kiss goodnight. When I looked at him, I asked if he felt okay. He said yes, and asked why. I told him his pupils were different sizes.

The next day he was in for an MRI. At one point the oncologist poked his head into the room and said he was waiting for the final read, but he thought that everything looked good and he'd be back in about ten minutes. He returned forty-five minutes later, and the look on his face said it all. Brian had several tiny tumors in his brain. They weren't causing his pupils to be different, but they were there. It was a day as devastating as his initial diagnosis almost five years earlier.

We tried several things including chemo and brain radiation, but nothing helped. The tumors kept growing. I look back at pictures of that summer, and though I didn't see it in person at the time, for the first time he looked sick. He looked like a cancer patient.

*

KATHIE SCOTT
Kathie's 57-year-old husband Jim
died from prostate cancer in 2009

I was prepared for the obvious changes of cancer such as hair loss or maybe weight loss. What I wasn't prepared for were the ones that weren't so obvious, such as bruising from bloodwork or treatments, and the side effects from certain chemo medicines. When we were in the middle of it, the changes were gradual and I didn't really see them. I just accepted the changes as part of the illness. Only in looking back can I see what cancer and the treatments did to him physically.

*

STEVE SHARP
Steve's 51-year-old wife Carolyn
died from melanoma in 2014

I spent considerable time researching the physical changes that someone would experience during their fight with cancer and the prescribed treatment. But that research was inadequate to prepare me for the sorrow and hopelessness I felt as I observed the effect cancer and it's treatment had on Carolyn.

My wife had beautiful curly hair which she lost in treatment. Before her struggle with cancer, she possessed an amazing intellect and memory. She had a masters in chemistry and was positively brilliant. Cancer robbed her of much of her cognitive ability and memory. These were the scariest changes, and I was helpless.

*

AUDRA THEROUX
Audra's father died from
esophageal cancer in 2014

I don't know if there is any way to ever be prepared for what cancer does to a loved one. You can read about it, people can tell you, but until you go through it yourself and see how it ravages someone you love, no words will ever fully prepare you. That, at least, was the case for me.

I've said before how I like knowledge. I researched everything and thought I understood what was going to happen to my dad. Until I saw it with my own eyes, nothing could have prepared me for not just the physical changes, but also the emotional changes. Cancer does not just change our loved one's body, it changes everything about who they are. That is by far the hardest part.

My dad had esophageal cancer so he lost a lot of weight. When he first got sick, he had extra weight to spare, so he never looked sickly or gaunt. Losing the weight actually looked good on him. He joked around about fitting into pants he hadn't fit into since he returned from Vietnam, and he wore them proudly even when dress pants might not be the appropriate dress code. The pants fit, right? He adamantly refused to go buy new jeans no matter how big all his pairs got on him. On days when he returned from chemotherapy with the med pack still clipped to his pants, I was afraid it would pull his pants down. I'd joke to him that no one wanted to see that, and it was probably time to go buy some new jeans. He never did, though. He kept wearing all his regular jeans and just kept tightening his belt.

If I hadn't been to all his appointments and saw his weights, his jeans and the extra skin on his neck would be how I would judge his weight loss. Looking back now, I don't think I realized just how much he physically changed, because I saw him every day. When I see pictures of him now, I realize just how skinny he got.

One picture in particular stands out in my mind. I found it in my phone after he died, and wondered who it was and why I took it. As I looked at it closer, I realized it was my father. I couldn't believe I didn't recognize him at first—he was so thin. He didn't even look ill in the picture, just a nice healthy weight. Again, he was lucky he started with some extra weight, otherwise he really would have been thin and sickly looking.

Like the weight loss, I didn't really notice much in the way of hair loss since Dad didn't have much to start, and he always kept it short. So that never was much of an issue.

*

DIANNE WEST
Dianne's husband Vern died from
multiple myeloma in 2010 at age 69

Vern was always active, so seeing him confined to a bed was difficult. He came out of the initial surgery unable to walk, so we had to get used to using a wheelchair right from the start. We knew he would need to be in a rehab facility for a while but we did not expect that it would be twelve weeks before he came home. He'd make some progress at rehab and then a GI bleed would send him back to the hospital for a week. He'd be back to rehab for three weeks and then a pulmonary embolism returned him to the hospital for three weeks. Back and forth.

It was very hard seeing him suffer through each new crisis. He became frustrated that he couldn't do things he normally would have done and that often affected his behavior toward me. The home health nurse explained that he did that because he knew I'd always be there for him and it was safe to let out all of his frustrations on me. It helped to know that this behavior was normal.

I eventually felt more like his mother than his wife. I understood that it could not be helped. It was what he needed. But I missed the intimacy we had before cancer.

The scariest times were when he had medication reactions. His personality changed. Or he had no idea where he was and imagined all sorts of odd things. I would receive phone calls from him in the middle of the night begging me to come because someone was in his room who wanted to harm him. Or we'd be watching a sporting event on TV in rehab and when it was over he would say he was ready to head to the car, truly thinking that we were actually there at the event. I had to bring these things up often with nurses and doctors, and remind them this was not Vern's normal behavior. They seemed to write it off as typical of an elderly, very sick, patient.

I finally got some help when a nurse who had previously cared for Vern in the hospital saw him at rehab. She called to ask what happened to him. I explained that I had been trying to convince the staff that something was very wrong. She stepped in, talked to the charge nurse and the doctor, and discovered it was a severe reaction to the sleep medication he was given each night, which I didn't know he was receiving. It frightens me now to think of others who are hospitalized without having anyone to serve as their advocate.

*

I keep dreaming of a future, a future with
a long and healthy life, not lived in the
shadow of cancer but in the light.

PATRICK SWAYZE
*

94

I keep dreaming of a future, a future with
a long and healthy life, not lived in the
shadow of cancer but in the light.

PATRICK SWAYZE
*

CHAPTER SIX

The Stigma of Cancer

There is no worse disease than ignorance.
-ANONYMOUS

Cancer often carries a stigma that the patient somehow brought it on by not taking better care of him or herself, or they aren't doing enough to treat the cancer. Others fear the cancer patient may somehow be contagious, or withdraw out of fear of not knowing what to say. Did you or your loved one encounter stigma related to the cancer?

*

JANICE DEL VECCHIO
Janice lost her husband Stephen to bile duct cancer in 2006 at age 47, and her second husband John to pancreatic cancer in 2013 at age 55

I did encounter stigma with both husbands. My first husband was a heavy smoker. I thought it was just a matter of time before he was diagnosed with lung cancer or some other lung related disease. He couldn't quit smoking and was on a nicotine patch until he died. Never, ever did I think he would die from a rare cancer.

95

My second husband quit smoking in his younger years and didn't always eat health, but I couldn't fault either one. God only knows why this happened to them. I have no idea if people we knew felt they would catch cancer, as no one ever made us feel that way. It wasn't until they died that I felt a shift in people's attitude toward me.

*

CYNTHIA HORACEK
Cynthia's husband Don died from
rectal cancer in 2010 at age 57

Fortunately, no. We had nothing but support from friends and family. The only time I felt stigma was when we were coming home from a doctor appointment one day and Don wanted Taco Bell. I was just happy he was eating, but my neighbor, upon learning Don was eating fast food said, "The idea is to keep him alive." That upset me.

*

MARGARET HUTSELL
Margaret's 77-year-old husband Tom
died from pancreatic cancer in 2016

Blessedly, we did not ever encounter any stigma regarding Tom's cancer. The few strangers in stores or restaurants who might have glanced our way and noticed he was dressed for a cool fall day in the heat of summer were not responded to and we lived our daily lives as always. The few who greeted us with a sad face or with a whiny voice inquired, "How are you feeling," were also responded to as normally as we were feeling. We hid no truths, spoke no lies, or shared stories to make others feel better.

Our family was amazing, each and every one of them. We talked about memories, our fears, and about future plans put on hold. We could, and would, talk about everything every time we were together.

"Hutsell Strong" became our motto. Every morning Tom sent our three kids a text message with a numerical indication of how he was feeling along with a thoughtful message for the day. His number was between one and ten, with ten being super good. His usual number was a seven, and we were all happy with that as long as he lived.

*

LYNN JORDAAN
Lynn's 58-year-old husband Johan
died from esophageal cancer in 2014

Johan smoked heavily all through his life. We did have a person try to lecture him on his lifestyle choice, but was effectively shut down. We were lucky in that no one pulled away, and seemed to gather around us more. There were always visits from coworkers or friends.

Johan chose not to do surgery, which brought up huge emotions for some people. It was hard to watch them try to brow beat Johan into changing his mind about this. He stood his ground, and doctors and friends soon learned it would do no good to keep talking about it. I felt it was Johan's body and his choice. The surgery proposed was not guaranteed to stop the cancer from progressing, so it was easy to sit with him in this decision.

*

GAIL MARCHESA
Gail's husband John died from
colon cancer in 2009 at age 55

Most of the time I was mad at John for not getting checked when he should have, but then learned to accept it.

*

HEATHER MCLAUGHLIN
Heather's 35-year-old husband Derek
died from colorectal cancer in 2013

We encountered some of this stigma. Derek was a well-known firefighter in the Charlotte area. He took decent care of himself, even if he hated to go to the doctor. We got some backlash from some who believed in Eastern medicine, who said Derek should go into pure oxygen chambers, drink specific pH water, eat specific herbs, and other things, but Derek didn't want to. We did have coworkers and friends who didn't know what to say, but we had friends close enough to us who would tell them to just sit with us or catch us up on their lives. The biggest thing was for us to feel included and not segregated by the cancer. Our friends generally did a good job with that.

*

SUE NOVA
Sue's husband Dana died from
lung cancer in 2012 at age 46

Oh, yes! Dana smoked; heck, we both did. So getting lung cancer was obviously his fault. I can't count the number of people who said exactly that! So many people demonized him because of it.

Also, I was sent many articles about high alkaline, no sugar, clinics in Mexico, and treatment that insurance wouldn't covered but was guaranteed to cure his cancer.

"If you really wanted to have him get better you would do...."

It made me so angry. Did these people, as well-meaning as they may have been, think I hadn't scoured the internet for any shred of hope? For any credible treatment? I was told by one friend that if I loved Dana, I would try anything. I should let some quack come into my home to read his energy and would, for a down payment of five hundred dollars, tell us if he could help. For an additional fee, he would let us know what to do. With his guidance, of course.

*

SHERYL POCHEL
Sheryl's husband Brian died from
pancreatic cancer in 2011 at age 43

Brian was a chiropractor. He owned and operated his own clinic. The hardest thing we had to deal with was the drop off of patients. I'm sure it was hard for some to see Brian working. I had patients tell me they felt bad having him adjust their back because they knew it hurt Brian. He was determined, though, to keep his practice going. He worked through his chemo treatments up until a year before he died, when he just couldn't physically do it.

That was hard.

*

KATHIE SCOTT
Kathie's 57-year-old husband Jim
died from prostate cancer in 2009

I don't recall anyone saying that Jim should have done anything different to have avoided cancer. We never experienced anyone who thought they could catch cancer by being around him. There were a few friends and some family who didn't come around because they didn't know what to say or do. I wish this had not been so, because Jim loved a room full of family and friends, and many of them just didn't come around.

*

STEVE SHARP
Steve's 51-year-old wife Carolyn
died from melanoma in 2014

I was blessed because I did not experience any of the usual cancer stigmas. Everyone I encountered was incredibly kind to us. However, in her final month of life, a technician referred to Carolyn as my mom. Cancer aged her.

*

AUDRA THEROUX
Audra's father died from
esophageal cancer in 2014

I can't say that my father encountered any cancer stigma that I saw. He was blessed to have great friends around him that were very supportive. My father did his best to continue acting as normal as possible, right up until the end. He did not want to be treated any differently, and quite frankly, I don't think he would have stood for that if anyone had tried to. Most of the attitude that was encountered along the way, I have to admit, came from my father himself. He was stubborn and sometimes just did not want to admit in any way that he was sick and that some things needed to change. The people around him were great.

*

DIANNE WEST
Dianne's husband Vern died from
multiple myeloma in 2010 at age 69

I never heard anyone blame Vern or I for all of the things that happened during his cancer journey, but it would not surprise me at all if those comments had been made. People let us down. Close friends disappeared. Some were there in the early months, but most just stopped coming by.

I'd hear, "We don't want to see him like that," but how would they know what Vern looked like since they never took the time to visit? While I really wanted to reply with a harsh comment, instead I just asked them to please call Vern if they didn't want to see him. But very few called. This was so hurtful for us both. We couldn't understand how they could just disappear when we needed them most. But when I brought this topic up with other caregivers, I learned it apparently is quite common. It's a real shame.

*

At times our own light goes out and is rekindled by
a spark from another person. Each of us has cause
to think with deep gratitude of those who have
lighted the flame within us.

ALBERT SCHWEITZER
*

CHAPTER SEVEN

The Financial Impact

Having cancer gave me membership in an elite
club I'd rather not belong to. -GILDA RADNER

Any chronic health condition can quickly take a financial toll on the family. The inability to work because of treatment, or lack of health insurance coupled with mounting medical bills can cause normal day-to-day expenses like groceries and gas feel pinched. How did the cancer affect your finances?

*

JANICE DEL VECCHIO
Janice lost her husband Stephen to bile duct cancer in 2006 at age 47,
and her second husband John to pancreatic cancer in 2013 at age 55

With both husbands, I was able to work full-time almost to the end of their lives. That was the way they wanted it. They wanted our normal life to stay the same as much as possible. I was fortunate that my employer was very understanding and flexible. Both husbands' employers kept them on health insurance and paid a hundred percent of it. I can never verbalize to them my appreciation of that.

It was a challenge to live on a reduced salary but we figured it out. The resource that was least helpful was support for the caregiver. There weren't many resources or support groups for that stage in my life. I sought out and attended one-on-one counseling on my own. It was also hard to take care of myself at that time. You put yourself on the shelf for an indeterminate amount of time.

*

CYNTHIA HORACEK
Cynthia's husband Don died from
rectal cancer in 2010 at age 57

My husband was a saver and managed our investments himself, so he left me well prepared to handle financial issues. However, I did not understand investing at all and hired a financial planner after his death. We were also among the lucky (if you can call it luck) who had excellent health insurance through Don's employer, and all his medical expenses were covered.

But I miss his help making decisions. That's probably one of the hardest things I deal with. "Can I afford this or not?" is a question I often ask myself. It's just a matter of not being financially astute. I had always imagined I'd be better than I am at handling money on my own. I didn't want to be dependent on someone to help me with this. It's something that I struggle with.

*

MARGARET HUTSELL
Margaret's 77-year-old husband Tom
died from pancreatic cancer in 2016

Tom had been retired nineteen years at the time of his diagnosis, and our finances were not jeopardized by his illness. Our supplemental insurance provider was exceptional to connect with and, combined with Medicare, paid for practically everything.

The only thing that caused us to say "What?!" was the cost of the dietary pancreatic enzymes we were told we needed for the first two to three months. Those were paid out of pocket and cost a thousand dollars each time we picked them up, which was every two weeks. We were happy our second oncologist finally told us we didn't need them since Tom still had his pancreas.

*

LYNN JORDAAN
Lynn's 58-year-old husband Johan
died from esophageal cancer in 2014

I count us extremely fortunate to live in Canada. All treatments were covered by Ontario Health Care. The company he was working for could not have been more supportive and did all they could not to disrupt our income. They arranged for disability insurance to be paid out. Canada Pension was paid out. All in all, our monthly finances were not affected.

*

GAIL MARCHESA
Gail's husband John died from
colon cancer in 2009 at age 55

I took family leave about a month and a half before John died, and he cashed in his 401(k), which was not a ton, so it would pay bills and keep us going for a while if we needed it. Again my problem came after, not because of life insurance.

*

HEATHER MCLAUGHLIN
Heather's 35-year-old husband Derek
died from colorectal cancer in 2013

The cancer affected our finances some, but we were very lucky to have an insurance that covered us once we met the low deductibles. Derek was the network manager for a private day school, and was the type of person who kept working until he had to give it up. They worked it out so Derek had one hundred percent coverage once he was on leave. This really helped us and we knew we were fortunate. The medication was expensive but again once we met our deductibles, we were okay.

We were also lucky in the fact that Derek's parents helped us with housing while he was getting five weeks of chemo and radiation in Atlanta, and then again in the hotel for a month and a half in Florida.

*

SUE NOVA
Sue's husband Dana died from
lung cancer in 2012 at age 46

Thankfully, our finances were impacted very little. We had long-term disability insurance. So aside from me losing some days here and there, we never lost insurance coverage or any of Dana's pay.

*

SHERYL POCHEL
Sheryl's husband Brian died from
pancreatic cancer in 2011 at age 43

As a young couple, our finances were never great. Just before his diagnosis, our clinic achieved all our financial goals. It was so exciting, we finally felt like we were getting where we needed to be. We had been in practice for just over five years. Even though we always had just enough for what we needed, it was nice to be able to project to our future and do some of the things we wanted to do.

Though we never relied on credit to survive, there were things that we did that I wish we hadn't. I worked for Brian in his clinic, and we often went without paychecks so we could pay our employees. Not paying Brian was one of the biggest mistakes we could have made. That lack of an actual paycheck means that the kids and I get very little in Social Security benefits. It is frustrating, for sure. He worked so hard to achieve his goals. He worked for eleven years as a chiropractor and what we get monthly is just enough to cover our basic bills, minus my mortgage.

On one hand, our lack of income was helpful because we qualified for our state Medicaid program. Brian was later given Social Security Disability, which then also put him on Medicare, so we never paid a medical bill. Not one. It would have financially devastated us if we had had to pay for his treatments and multiple surgeries. If we had not had that, I know Brian would not have fought as hard as he did to survive. He never would have left me with an insurmountable debt.

*

KATHIE SCOTT
Kathie's 57-year-old husband Jim
died from prostate cancer in 2009

In some ways we were very lucky, and in others not so. My job carried the medical insurance for us and it never let us down and never questioned any treatments, they just paid. Unfortunately, when Jim had to stop working, our income was cut considerably and Social Security Disability couldn't completely make up for it. Most of our savings and retirement fund disappeared, but I would do nothing differently in that respect. I never wanted to deny him or us anything we wanted or anywhere we wanted to go during his illness.

Jim had been self-employed all his working life and we had finally hit our financial stride, so to speak, but cancer brought all of those plans to a screeching halt. I can't really say we had outside resources helping us. Neither of us were very good at asking for help so we just managed on our own for the most part.

*

STEVE SHARP
Steve's 51-year-old wife Carolyn
died from melanoma in 2014

Because of good decisions made before Carolyn was diagnosed with cancer, the disease did not impact our finances. Because we had lost our previous spouses, we understood the necessity of having good health and disability insurance. Once she was diagnosed with stage IV melanoma, she immediately starting receiving payments from both work and Social Security Disability. We were blessed to have all of my wife's cancer expenses covered. My employer allowed me to work part time and still keep my benefits while Carolyn underwent treatment, and allowed me to take a month off after Carolyn's death.

The local hospice provided tremendous help by contributing feedback on critical decisions.

*

AUDRA THEROUX
Audra's father died from
esophageal cancer in 2014

Cancer is expensive. My father had two insurance plans at the time of his diagnosis, and still managed to rack up insured medical bills during the seven months he had cancer. Because he was retired at the time he became ill, it did not affect his job at all. Had he been working at the time, there is no way he could have continued to work. He had chemotherapy and doctor appointments weekly, and when he started radiation, that was daily. Not to mention, the hospital where he was being treated was in Massachusetts and we live in New Hampshire, so we traveled to get there and receive better care.

I was not working at the time my father became ill, due to my own health complications. Prior to his cancer, he took care of me, and drove me to and from the hospital. When he became sick, we did a complete role reversal. My being out of work allowed me to devote my time to my father and his health. I don't know what I would have done if I had been working. I needed to be there with him, and I am so blessed and thankful I had those seven months with him.

We never took advantage of any resources for him. From the time of my father's diagnosis to the time of his passing was so fast, we never had time to think about resources or what he might need. He had two insurance plans and the bills hadn't started to pile in until after he passed away.

*

DIANNE WEST
Dianne's husband Vern died from
multiple myeloma in 2010 at age 69

We were quite lucky to have good insurance. I had always carried my husband on my work insurance plan because it was cheaper than his teacher insurance. He turned sixty-five just before his diagnosis, so he was covered by Medicare. We had my insurance as a supplement and he also had some coverage from his work for the arena. Our out-of-pocket expenses were manageable because we were using plan providers. I do recall being shocked when the first Explanation of

Benefits statement arrived from the hospital. Over eight hundred thousand dollars for a two-week stay and two surgeries! I never did total everything up, but at one point we had reached three million dollars in charges. I am so very grateful we had insurance coverage.

I had to move into a different job due to the amount of time I needed to take off to care for Vern. It was not handled well and I was terribly hurt by my boss and some coworkers' behaviors. However, it ended up being a blessing to move into a position where I could tele-commute, and I was grateful to still have a job with a good income and insurance. One less thing to worry about.

Vern's employer, a casino, let him go the month following his diagnosis when it became obvious he was not going to be able to return to work in the foreseeable future.

*

I'm not searching for the meaning of life, but
I'm looking for a meaning within my life.

DAVID LOWERY
*

CHAPTER EIGHT

Caring For Our Loved One

There's this whole mythology that people bravely
battle their cancer and then they become
survivors. Well, the ones who don't survive
may be just as brave, just as courageous.
-BARBARA EHRENREICH

Caring for a loved one with cancer can be a sacred time full of love. Other times it can feel emotionally overwhelming and too much to handle. In your experience, what was it like caring for a loved one with cancer?

*

JANICE DEL VECCHIO
Janice lost her husband Stephen to bile duct cancer in 2006 at age 47, and her second husband John to pancreatic cancer in 2013 at age 55

I took care of two terminally ill spouses. When my second husband became ill, it was like I had crossed into a vortex that had me living my life over. I was stunned that I was going through this again.

Initially it was hard for me to be the cheerleader. I felt I had to keep it together, not cry, not complain and most of all be positive. I went to every doctor appointment they had. A good day was when my husbands felt good enough to get out and enjoy a beautiful day, go for dinner, take a walk on the beach, or go away overnight. Bad days were when they were too sick to get out of bed or they were overcome with emotion as to what was happening to them. Learning to listen instead of trying to figure out the answers for why our world was suddenly turned upside down was difficult. Terminally ill patients often suffer from depression and I made it my mission to try to stay on top of it. I was scared for them and me. On bad days, I would go outside and take a walk or arrange to have a lunch or dinner with a friend. I found a therapist for myself and it was great to have someone with no vested interest to talk to. It was my no judgment zone.

My salvation was that I was able to continue to work full-time during both husbands illnesses. My employer was very sympathetic to what was going on and the pressure that was on me. When my husbands were hospitalized, I was still able to work, as the hospitals were in same city. The hospital staff had all my contact information and often encouraged me to get out of the building for a bit. I often went to a restaurant near the hospital for dinner and a couple glasses of wine. This was thirty minutes to escape all that was happening. I look back and wonder how I managed to survive. You just do what you have to get through the day and, basically, you don't think about what is going on while it is happening.

*

CYNTHIA HORACEK
Cynthia's husband Don died from
rectal cancer in 2010 at age 57

A good day was when Don was feeling okay—not sick. A bad day was having to go to the emergency room, or when he was passing out from low blood pressure, usually from bleeding. Or when the surgeon told me he couldn't remove the entire tumor. That was scary—I knew it only took one cell to spread. I stopped working to care for him, and over time I worried about not bringing in money. He reassured me that he his disability insurance would pay his full salary.

A bad day was when I was frightened and wanted to protect him from my fears but didn't want to burden him with not having hope. And we both had hope; we were sure he would beat this. It was hard caring for him, but I wouldn't have it any other way. I think loving someone means sometimes doing things that are unpleasant, like caring for them when they get ill. I know he would have done the same thing for me.

*

MARGARET HUTSELL
Margaret's 77-year-old husband Tom
died from pancreatic cancer in 2016

I felt tired, stress was always present, and I worried about getting though each day without a trip to the emergency room. I worried about what laid ahead, and worried about keeping my husband's spirits up. My own emotions bounced around constantly.

Having said all of the above, taking care of Tom was an honor, a privilege and I would have done anything, at any time, to make his cancer journey pain-free and peaceful.

We talked about everything that was on our minds. It didn't matter what the subject matter was, we were able to share our hearts and thoughts without holding anything back.

A good day was a normal day. Tom would get up and shower, and fix us both a bite of breakfast. We did his daily tube irrigation and made sure dressings were clean and tape wasn't pulling anything. He would go outside in his yard with a cup of coffee and walk the yard checking on his plants and shrubs. If he felt good enough (and, he did feel good enough until two weeks before his death) he would putter outside as long as he could, breathing in the fresh air and getting his hands and knees dirty, and smile the entire time.

We'd have a bite of supper and watch a bit of TV or share a bottle of wine and talk some more. Reaching for my hand at bedtime was the one new addition to our routine. Every night, he reached for my hand to hold. I held on for dear life. We knew what was ahead, but had no idea what was really coming. Holding hands made it feel okay.

*

LYNN JORDAAN
Lynn's 58-year-old husband Johan
died from esophageal cancer in 2014

Caring for Johan was the hardest, most rewarding thing I have ever done. In the beginning, he was very resilient and didn't really need caring for, aside from the occasional reminder of an upcoming appointment or to take meds. Toward the end, we had hospice nurses coming in once or twice a day to change pain meds and monitor him. I quickly became familiar with how to change IV bags and prime the automatic med dispenser, thus eliminating a middle of the night visit from the nurse, which was disturbing to all of us. He started calling me Nurse Ratched.

On good days there was much laughter, albeit with a slight undertone of sadness. On bad days, it was grin and bear it, get through this next thing, tomorrow may be a little better. Long walks and quick shopping trips were my recharge times. Thank the good Lord for hospice volunteers. It was still hard to leave him, knowing that the end was near and wanting to get all the time with him I could before he died. But I knew that in order to give him my best, I had to care for me too. I also found I could cry in the shower, and no one would hear.

*

GAIL MARCHESA
Gail's husband John died from
colon cancer in 2009 at age 55

It was frustrating at times because I tried to help by making sure meds were taken, and trying to get food down John was very hard. Then the doctor's visits were not fun because he would ask me why and why not. On good days, John would get up and do a few things before he wore out. Some days he would take a bath (was afraid he would fall in shower) and lay on the bed for the next couple of hours.

*

HEATHER MCLAUGHLIN
Heather's 35-year-old husband Derek
died from colorectal cancer in 2013

Caring for Derek was different every day. Since his type of cancer did not respond to treatment very well, and he had just about every side effect one could have, when we called his oncologist to ask a question about something, the answer was always, "go to the hospital." It got old for me, and very frustrating for Derek. We spent countless hours in the waiting room, on the cancer floor, in testing rooms, you name it. Eventually, Derek didn't want me to call and update the doctor because we knew the answer. He would get angry and punch the wall. He threw a glass at the wall once and it shattered. He apologized; he never put me in harm's way, but you never knew what the cancer was going to do.

As for food, Derek would get a craving and I would go get the food but then his appetite would change or he would get nauseous, or he wouldn't know what he wanted so he would order a lot of food. If I cooked in the house, which wasn't often, the lingering smell would make him nauseous. I hated it. The constant nausea meds that didn't work were just one more facet of the cancer that took over Derek.

Derek would forget things. He wanted to drive, but knowing the amount of meds he was on, I couldn't let him. He would get up from his recliner and get dizzy and fall. That was the worst, having the fight or flight response kick in and having to pick him up again and then make sure he was okay. One time, he fell down the stairs trying to answer the door I had accidentally locked. Derek told me that one of our dogs, Rio, a Belgian Malinois, helped him get up. An amazing dog.

With all the struggles of caring for Derek, over the final three to four months, he was really only awake for a couple of hours in the afternoon. It was then when he was most like Derek. We could have a few conversations about what our life had been, had become, and what it would like in the future. Derek could tell me he loved me, and I could tell him I loved him.

*

SUE NOVA
Sue's husband Dana died from
lung cancer in 2012 at age 46

Caring for someone, my beautiful husband who had cancer, was so many things. Obviously, it was scary and painful but it was also beautiful. We developed an intimacy that only comes, I think, from seeing each other at their most fragile, scared, and vulnerable. We spoke of things that we hadn't ever thought we would have to. I saw things and did things, for him, that a wife shouldn't have to do. I call cancer the most beautiful horrible thing.

In the beginning, it was different. I thought he should try harder to participate in life, eat more, or to eat, period. I got my feelings hurt if he didn't want to eat what I had cooked. Unfortunately, I lashed out at him and complained to others. I don't know when that changed, but it did. We began to have much more open dialogues. I went on FMLA because there was no way he could stay home alone.

I will say that it was the most difficult thing I had ever done. I was constantly on alert to his movements. If he got out of bed and began wandering without his walker. What if he tried to go to the bathroom unassisted? What if something happened in the middle of the night? I lived on a few hours of sleep, nervous energy, and coffee. To say I was tired is an understatement.

*

SHERYL POCHEL
Sheryl's husband Brian died from
pancreatic cancer in 2011 at age 43

Caring for a cancer patient brings all kinds of emotions to the surface. Since Brian was a doctor, he was extremely knowledgeable about the body, but that didn't make him the easiest person to deal with. I spent hours every day researching his cancer and the treatments that were available.

I will say that most of our days were good. We both lived with hope and knew that even though cancer was part of our life, it wasn't the whole thing. However, Brian did suffer from depression, and the cancer diagnosis and treatments didn't help. There were days when he was short with us, and sometimes even mean. Those days were not common, but they were there. It frustrated me that he wouldn't do anything to try to improve that situation. He said therapy and antidepressants wouldn't change the fact that he had cancer.

When it came to me, my needs were often put on the back burner. I was taking care of Brian, our four young kids, and making sure his clinic stayed running when he couldn't be there. There was no time in my day to recharge myself. It has taken me years to recharge from his cancer, and I am just now in a place where I feel truly whole.

*

KATHIE SCOTT
Kathie's 57-year-old husband Jim
died from prostate cancer in 2009

Caring for a loved one who is sick is both difficult and rewarding. Watching someone you love deteriorate before your eyes while you are helpless to make it stop is so heartbreaking. Sometimes all of the days seemed bad, but when we would go to the doctor and get a positive lab or scan result, it was like winning the lottery! We couldn't wait to get out of the office and make those wonderful phone calls with positive news. When the results were not great, it was as if you were trying to pull a tractor trailer behind you. The weight of bad news was unbearable. My friend's husband passed away suddenly several years prior to our meeting and she was a huge support system for me. She told me that losing her husband was the worst thing she could imagine but she couldn't fathom what it would have been like to watch him die over a span of years. She was my battery charger.

*

STEVE SHARP
Steve's 51-year-old wife Carolyn
died from melanoma in 2014

Caring for someone with cancer is akin to have ridden an emotional rollercoaster with many ups and down. There were times when we thought that Carolyn had beat her cancer only to be told a short time later that she was terminal.

Carolyn would have days without pain, where she could find something about which to laugh or smile. These were good days. Then there were bad days in which she experienced terrible headaches from the tumors in her brain. On these days, Carolyn would asleep, and I would pray that God would be merciful. Sometimes I would spend a half hour by myself on my spinning bike just to take my mind off of Carolyn's struggle. It helped me cope.

*

DIANNE WEST
Dianne's husband Vern died from
multiple myeloma in 2010 at age 69

I felt honored to be able to care for Vern. It was a physical example of our marriage vows. But it was hard, hard work. There are emotional issues seeing your loved one going through this and there are physical issues with the actual heavy lifting required. I found that it became my identity, and I'm not sure that was a good thing.

Good days were when Vern would wake up, bright-eyed and ready to face the day. We'd have great conversations. He'd watch his sports on TV. We'd laugh. He'd eat well. We might even take a drive to Red Rock or out to Lake Mead. It would be like before, except for the hospital bed, the PICC line, the hemodialysis lines, the colostomy bag, the wheelchair. We didn't get a lot of these days, unfortunately. Well, perhaps that's not true. During the year of his partial remission there were good days. It's just that those days seem to have disappeared from my memory after the very difficult final eighteen months.

Bad days were when I had trouble waking him and he would fight with me about having to eat or get ready for dialysis or a chemo appointment. When he didn't want to get up out of his bed or his recliner. When I could see how tired he was of all that he was having to deal with.

Really bad days were when he was running a temperature or his blood pressure dropped really low, or he started bleeding and I knew we'd be heading back to the hospital once again.

While I hated it whenever he had to return to the hospital, those days did allow me to recharge a bit. Someone else was responsible for his care and I was able to breathe easier. I could keep watch and be his advocate, but the whole responsibility didn't land on my shoulders.

*

Slow progress is still progress.

LYNDA CHELDELIN FELL
*

CHAPTER NINE

Caregiving Options

Caregiving often calls us to lean into love
we didn't know possible. – TIA WALKER

Giving care to someone we love is natural, but caregiving is the role of providing constant physical and emotional support to a patient. Caregivers take on necessary duties such as driving to treatment, arranging medical appointments, and providing needed care and emotional support. In many cases, they also take on many of the roles formerly handled by the person who has been diagnosed. Were you the main caregiver for your loved one, or did you hire a family member or outside help?

*

JANICE DEL VECCHIO
Janice lost her husband Stephen to bile duct cancer in 2006 at age 47, and her second husband John to pancreatic cancer in 2013 at age 55

I was the main caregiver for both husbands. Both agreed we would make all the decisions together as long as we could. I believe this experience brought us to a deeper love and understanding. We were both crushed by what was happening and we supported each other. I was the main caretaker because I was the only one who would do it. I had help from family (mostly mine) on a regular basis but all of the responsibility fell to me. Both husbands were in awe and appreciated everything I did for them. They were both worried about me and what would happen to me once they were gone. It was very sweet and moving. They would defend me if someone criticized me or questioned the care they were receiving. We were a team.

*

CYNTHIA HORACEK
Cynthia's husband Don died from
rectal cancer in 2010 at age 57

I was the main caregiver for my husband. For most of the period he was ill, he didn't need a lot of care, beyond driving him to radiation and chemo and doctor appointments. When he first had his tumor removed, he was on TPN (total parenteral nutrition) and I had to hook him up each night and unhook him in the mornings. I was fearful of doing this because everything had to be kept sterile and very clean, but I learned quickly and was able to do this without a problem. After the tumor was removed, he had an ostomy and I helped him change the bag for several weeks before he was comfortable changing it himself. Fortunately, I'm not squeamish. And again, it's one of those things you do for someone you love. If anything I think my caring for my husband made us closer and stronger.

*

MARGARET HUTSELL
Margaret's 77-year-old husband Tom
died from pancreatic cancer in 2016

I was all he had and, more importantly, all he wanted. I learned how to administer shots in his tummy when blood clots formed in his lungs due to chemo. I irrigated his biliary catheter twice daily and, for the first three months emptied his bag of bile. Toward the end, I learned how to drain ascites from a tube, and on and on. Meds were checked off, food intake was journaled, and when the shaking and fevers came on, I covered him with three blankets, a wool hat on his head, and held his hand till they abated. Or I would bundle him up and take him to the emergency room.

Tom was always telling me how grateful he was that I was willing to care for him in these various duties. I always responded with the same phrase. "I love you and it is an honor to be here for you." We were completely connected throughout the entire fourteen months of his illness. We often said it was such a gift and seemed like icing on the cake, because we did it together—strangely so, but true. We focused only on each other, did only what we wanted to do, and only with people we wanted to be with.

*

LYNN JORDAAN
Lynn's 58-year-old husband Johan
died from esophageal cancer in 2014

I was the main caregiver. I had help from my daughter when she came home over the weekends, and toward the end I had called in hospice and had a volunteer look in periodically. The decision for Johan to stay at home was taken together, the hospice help was taken by me. It did strain things a bit until I explained that the volunteer was coming in for my own peace of mind. He felt he didn't need anyone to watch over him when he was just sleeping anyway. I was worried he would die alone, so as in any marriage, we came to a compromise. The volunteer wouldn't have to be in the bedroom if he was sleeping but would be available if things went south.

*

GAIL MARCHESA
Gail's husband John died from
colon cancer in 2009 at age 55

We decided I would take family leave, and he was going to cash in some benefits he had. That would keep everything going for about three months. After two months or so, we got hospice because John didn't want to come back to the hospital anymore. We had hospice for two weeks before he died. They were the best.

*

HEATHER MCLAUGHLIN
Heather's 35-year-old husband Derek
died from colorectal cancer in 2013

I was the main caregiver for Derek. Family members and friends came to help out for a couple hours here and there, but it was me and him fighting head-on. I would say this did put a strain on our relationship because everything was on me. Derek asked me to do things that should not be asked of a wife, but I know, and knew then too, it was the cancer talking. When we would go out or when we went on our final trip to England, I was scared out of my mind. It was me who knew all the medicine dosages, what should and shouldn't go together, how his body reacted to certain things. I was his person. I was the person who stood up for him.

*

SUE NOVA
Sue's husband Dana died from
lung cancer in 2012 at age 46

I was the primary caregiver for my husband. There were a couple of reasons for this. Mainly it was because he would get agitated if I wasn't around. I was the only one he would allow to go into the bathroom with him, shower him, and give him his meds. I was, also, one of the only people who understood him, as he was losing his ability to communicate. Also, none of our family lived close by. That was their excuse. That includes his mom and brother. No one volunteered to come be with him. I think it was because they felt uncomfortable being in the presence of someone who was dying. I could be wrong, but I don't think I am.

Our oldest daughter came out when she could, which was mostly weekends. She was juggling school, marriage, and a one-hundred-mile drive. The only time I really got any substantial help was when my oldest daughter called hospice and let them know they needed to come help me or I would likely snap. That came in the form of round-the-clock nursing only for the last two weeks of his life.

*

SHERYL POCHEL
Sheryl's husband Brian died from
pancreatic cancer in 2011 at age 43

I was Brian's caregiver. I rarely asked anyone for help. He was MY husband, MY best friend, my everything. In many ways I believe that this brought us closer than we had ever been. I was the one person in Brian's life that he truly trusted and I wouldn't have done anything differently. Toward the end it was harder as we had moved from a partnership to patient/caregiver roles. The intimacy that had once been so prevalent in our relationship was all but gone. That hurt, but the love was still there and strong. It is still there and just as strong.

We never got any outside help until the end of his life when I made the decision to have him moved from the hospital to hospice. I didn't want him dying at home. I couldn't deal with that. Hospice was an amazing thing and the best choice I could have made. Those two weeks were hard, but the care he received was second to none.

*

KATHIE SCOTT
Kathie's 57-year-old husband Jim
died from prostate cancer in 2009

I was the only caregiver. In my mind, nobody could do it like I could so asking for help was not an option. My family would offer to go to doctor appointments with him but I knew they just wouldn't ask the right questions or be able to relay information correctly. My husband didn't offer any opinions on my caregiver status but in the beginning he did go to a few appointments and even some chemo treatments alone. This was what he wanted. I knew he probably just needed some space and to feel he wasn't a burden.

*

STEVE SHARP
Steve's 51-year-old wife Carolyn
died from melanoma in 2014

Because we had a number of family and friends available, we all shared in Carolyn's caregiving and functioned as a team. This was important as I continued to work during this time to maintain our health insurance. My friends understood that and were incredibly supportive. My wife and I agreed on this together, yet it was very hard for her to accept that she could no longer do things for herself such as driving to appointments, preparing meals, and being independent. Because of her frustration, she would lash out at close family members, which was not like her at all.

And, as wonderful as all the help was at the time, it did make it harder for us to have private time to have the conversations that we needed to have.

*

DIANNE WEST
Dianne's husband Vern died from
multiple myeloma in 2010 at age 69

I was Vern's sole caregiver. I never thought about hiring anyone to help, as it felt like this was part of my life's purpose. Vern and I married just two-and-a-half months after our first date and it always seemed that our paths were meant to cross at exactly that moment. When he became ill and needed such heavy care, those feelings returned. This. This is why we had found one another. He needed me.

We had a weekly visit from a home healthcare nurse early on, but I was eventually trained to flush and change the bandages on his PICC line, to give him those belly shots he hated, to hang an IV when he needed to be on antibiotics for several weeks, to clean and bandage the pressure ulcer, to change out his colostomy bag. Vern relied on me being there to take care of his needs. He trusted me.

I did have a couple of people I could ask to sit with him if I needed to go into the office or to the grocery store during those times when he couldn't be left alone. I could always count on his friend Joe to come over when needed and our son Jeremy was often there to keep an eye on his dad.

*

CHAPTER TEN

The Support Circle

Never believe that a few caring people can't
change the world. For indeed, that's all
we ever have. – MARGARET MEAD

Families and cancer are complicated. The unique dynamics that define each family can be precarious in challenging times, leaving caregivers hesitant to delegate support. Others aren't comfortable asking for assistance, and eschew outside help. Did you allow family and friends to provide secondary help such a meals, errands, and respite?

*

JANICE DEL VECCHIO
Janice lost her husband Stephen to bile duct cancer in 2006 at age 47,
and her second husband John to pancreatic cancer in 2013 at age 55

I took as much help as I could get. I would have loved for someone to help out with meals, but no one offered. My family was great about going to treatment appointments for my first husband. It gave me a break and I was able to go to work. My family helped out with my second husband by offering emotional support to me. They didn't know John, my second husband, as well as my first. John and I were only together for two years.

My advice to anyone who is a caregiver is to take time for yourself. Get professional counseling if you feel you need it. Don't be afraid to ask someone for help. Most people want to help but don't know what you need. If you need help with food or housekeeping, ask. Most folks would be happy to help in any way they can. It empowers them as they feel they are doing something to help out. If you encounter anyone who is resistant to help, just move on. Not everyone can cope with illness or they just don't want to get involved. Though it is hard to not let it bother you.

*

CYNTHIA HORACEK
Cynthia's husband Don died from
rectal cancer in 2010 at age 57

I welcomed meals from friends. I welcomed support and help from my family, except it wasn't really needed for the year he was sick. It was after his death that I needed the extra love, help, and support. But I appreciated anything anyone did for us. My parents lived much closer to the hospital and chemo center when he had treatment and we would stay with them when he had appointments. When he had a hospital stay, I'd stay with them because they lived so close to the hospital. My father was a physician and it helped me a lot to having him nearby to offer me hope, and also the reality of what we were facing was easy to discuss with him.

*

MARGARET HUTSELL
Margaret's 77-year-old husband Tom
died from pancreatic cancer in 2016

Occasionally, family would offer to bring suppers, but Tom's appetite was so varied, that soon stopped. Our friends never offered and neighbors stayed away, except for one couple who did help with mowing the grass and came to visit occasionally. I suggest asking for what you need and doing only what you can do for each other. Let the small stuff go and lean on those you are comfortable with.

*

LYNN JORDAAN
Lynn's 58-year-old husband Johan
died from esophageal cancer in 2014

I didn't really have a lot of offers for errands, etc. I did have a close friend who brought meals, and I had hospice when I really needed it.

I think we have always been self-sufficient so it didn't really occur to me to reach out. I did have my daughter move back home for the last couple of weeks of Johan's life, more so that she could spend some quality time with her dad than anything else.

I would advise people embarking on this journey to make use of every service available. Take care of yourselves first (there is a reason they say fit the mask on your own face first in airplanes) and remember to breathe. Looking after someone who has cancer is hard work: physically, emotionally and spiritually.

*
GAIL MARCHESA
Gail's husband John died from
colon cancer in 2009 at age 55

My girlfriend was there a lot. I never refused help, so I was lucky there. My journey is not over, yet I discover different things as I go and some I am proud of because they are independent which I never thought I was. I am not lonely most times but every once in a while, yes. When things happen out of the ordinary, I just figure John is up to something and he's with all of our fur kids who passed.

*

HEATHER MCLAUGHLIN
Heather's 35-year-old husband Derek
died from colorectal cancer in 2013

In the beginning, we thought we could do it all. During the five weeks of chemo and radiation in Atlanta, it wasn't until about halfway through that I got bogged down in grading and my mother-in-law offered to help grade. That was a huge help. She also helped with the dogs and cleaned the house for me so I didn't have to worry about it.

During the surgery in Florida, I let friends take care of our house. There was no way I could be in Florida and North Carolina at the same time. Family brought food to me in Derek's room to make sure I ate, so that was good, too.

In November 2012, just before Thanksgiving, one of the assistant principals at the school I was teaching at sat me down and told me to call Joe and to give her the phone. The conversation went as follows.

"Joe, can you take over Heather's classes starting tomorrow?"

Joe says sure. Sharon says great. End of conversation.

I had already worked it out with Joe, since he was a chemistry teacher too. See, Sharon had known because I told her and a few others that Derek was only really awake for a few hours in the afternoon. In a mom's voice that only moms can do, she told me to go be with Derek before he dies so I can spend quality time with him. And that was the end of it that day in her office. I couldn't have been working for a better administration or with a better science department. They surrounded me with love during my entire time there.

This is also when the fire department started dropping by more just to say hi, or see if we needed anything. If they didn't stop by, I got texts. We felt loved. I would encourage people facing it now to not push out their friends. Have a list of stuff that needs to be done, even if it seems stupid. Get milk, pick up dog food, mail letters, mow the lawn, etc. for friends to do if they want. It can even be something as small as take the kids for thirty minutes, take the dogs for a walk, or sit with my husband while I do this. I found friends want to help, they just don't know how.

*

SUE NOVA
Sue's husband Dana died from
lung cancer in 2012 at age 46

The only true assistance I got was in the form of meals. The church we attended had a rotating schedule of people who cooked meals for us and either leave them at the church or come drop them off. On the weekends my daughter did the shopping if we needed anything. Or she and her husband would stay with Dana while I went to the store. That was less likely to happen, as he could sense I was gone and would get upset. Sometimes on the weekends, my daughter came over and I would try to nap.

Again, it wasn't a matter of allowing people to help. It's that mostly they just didn't or wouldn't.

*

SHERYL POCHEL
Sheryl's husband Brian died from
pancreatic cancer in 2011 at age 43

We did have friends and family bring us meals and help care for the kids. Brian's cancer was a five and a half-year journey and we had an initial outpouring of meals and gifts. We even had someone doing our laundry, which was amazing given we were a family of six with four young ones. In the in-between years when Brian had no evidence of disease, all that ceased and we just lived life.

In 2011, when cancer spread to his brain, we again had people helping with meals and laundry. I did let some people take Brian to various appointments, but for the most part I did it all. He was my person.

The one piece of advice I have for people who are now faced with this kind of situation is to make a list. What do you need? What do you want? What errands need to be done? Housework? Meals?

Running the kids here and there? Yardwork? Home repairs? WRITE THEM ALL DOWN! When someone offers to help, give them the list and ask what can they do? What can they help with?

I know most people were sincere with their offers, but they don't know what to do, and the problem is that our heads are spinning and we don't know what we need. Making a list gives people something concrete and allows them to pick something that fits with their schedule and abilities.

*

KATHIE SCOTT
Kathie's 57-year-old husband Jim
died from prostate cancer in 2009

I felt like I managed most things without help. People would occasionally say "Let me know what I can do," but I was never comfortable asking. One friend knew I was having trouble making time for regular haircuts so she rounded up a hairdresser who came to my house when we needed a group cut. This was done several times and it became a bit of a social event for me to see some friends and have people in the house. I am forever grateful to her.

If you are in the cancer journey, ask for help and accept all offers of help. Do not try to do this alone, call in your markers. Talk to your spouse about important things such as money and funeral arrangements. Most of all, talk about your life—the good and the bad.

*

STEVE SHARP
Steve's 51-year-old wife Carolyn
died from melanoma in 2014

As I stated before, we were blessed to have family and friends provide transportation to medical appointments, run errands, provide meals and spend time with Carolyn so I could do other things that needed to be done.

One friend set up a website to coordinate care and other activities for us. This was incredibly helpful to have someone organize things because the primary caregiver is often so stressed that they are not always thinking clearly about the details.

*

DIANNE WEST
Dianne's husband Vern died from
multiple myeloma in 2010 at age 69

Vern had a good friend who was wonderfully helpful to both of us. Joe was one of the very, very few who stayed by our side the entire time. But he took it further than just being there. He spent quality time with Vern whether he was at home, in the hospital, or at a rehab facility. They watched sports and, since they had worked together, he shared news of things that were happening at the arena. Joe made it possible for me to go into work and not have to leave Vern alone. And Joe showed up along with my friend Debbie right after we signed the papers for Vern to transfer from the hospital to hospice. Such divine inspiration for the two of them to appear when they did.

We were overloaded with food the first couple of weeks and then it stopped. A couple of my work friends came over and cleaned up our landscaping, which was a really thoughtful gift. Others brought over a Thanksgiving meal. But for the most part we felt very abandoned after the first couple of months.

People would say the standard, "Let me know if you need anything," but few caregivers are able to do that. We're juggling so many things we may not even know what we need. I've never been good at asking for help, so you would think my friends would know that. But they saw me handling it all—caring for Vern and going to work—and they assumed I had everything under control. I did not.

My recommendation for others who are facing a cancer journey is to ask a good friend to step in and just do it for you. Tell them what you need, or think you may need, and let them organize it. I've seen this talked about on Facebook. And there are even apps where people can sign up for when they'll provide a meal or run an errand or do some yardwork. What a blessing that would have been during those really hard times. And remind your person that this isn't just needed at the beginning of the journey. It's needed during the hard days that will arrive later. Leave a bouquet of flowers on the doorstep, drop off a special treat like coffee, donuts or home-baked cookies. When they're in the hospital, pick up the mail, take care of the yard, and visit. Oh, how I wish his friends would have taken just a few minutes out of their day to visit with him throughout the cancer years.

How people treat you is their karma;
how you react is yours.

WAYNE DYER
*

142

How people treat you is their karma;
how you react is yours.

WAYNE DYER

CHAPTER ELEVEN

Impact on Relationships

I know of no higher fortitude than stubbornness
in the face of overwhelming odds.
-LOUIS NIZER

Cancer doesn't affect just the person who was diagnosed. It touches relationships and family dynamics in unexpected ways. For some, facing and walking the journey together can strengthen a bond. For others, uncertainty about the future can bring about strain. How did the cancer affect your relationship with your loved one?

*

JANICE DEL VECCHIO
Janice lost her husband Stephen to bile duct cancer in 2006 at age 47,
and her second husband John to pancreatic cancer in 2013 at age 55

Well the biggest shift with both of my experiences with losing a spouse was the new caregiver role. Both husbands were fairly independent and struggled with having to depend on me for basic needs they were no longer able to do. I would have to say being a caregiver was the toughest job I ever had. It was constant stress, worry and feeling overwhelmed. What helped with my sanity was the fact I could still work full-time during their illnesses. Not a lot of folks are fortunate to be able to do that. I never had any disagreements with either of them on their treatment or care. Family members felt it was necessary to voice their opinions. We just ignored what we could. We worked as a team to make decisions of what was the best course of treatment and care.

*

CYNTHIA HORACEK
Cynthia's husband Don died from
rectal cancer in 2010 at age 57

I think that having cancer affects a relationship any way you look at it. There's the fear you get when you don't know what's going to happen, and not wanting to tell your partner how scared you are because you don't want him or her to be burdened with your fear, and you don't want to make it worse for them.

I think our relationship was strengthened because we were in it together; I wasn't going to let him deal with it alone. We didn't disagree about his care or treatment. The only thing I questioned was whether he was getting the best care possible or if we should have gone to a cancer treatment center, like the City of Hope for example. But we had good doctors and I know he had good treatment.

*

MARGARET HUTSELL
Margaret's 77-year-old husband Tom
died from pancreatic cancer in 2016

Tom's cancer made us stronger than we had ever been. We felt more love in those fourteen months than we had in a long time. We were married for fifty-six-plus years and were, indeed, joined at the hip. We had enjoyed nineteen years of his retirement and spent most of it at home doing things that needed doing and just being together.

We always considered our options with regard to his treatment plan. We would discuss with each other, do research on our laptops and share concerns with the medical care team as well as our kids. Disagreements were not part of our equation.

*

LYNN JORDAAN
Lynn's 58-year-old husband Johan
died from esophageal cancer in 2014

Cancer did not have a profound effect on our relationship, it was more a case of okay, another hurdle we face together. There was no disagreement about treatment per se, there was a bit of a hang up when I wanted hospice volunteers to come in. Johan didn't want strangers around. I had to be firm and explain that the volunteers weren't actually there for him, but to help give me peace of mind. He reluctantly agreed.

*

GAIL MARCHESA
Gail's husband John died from
colon cancer in 2009 at age 55

We did get closer because that was all that was left of being normal. At times, I felt very resentful having to do everything but kept my mouth shut and it went away after a bit.

*

HEATHER MCLAUGHLIN
Heather's 35-year-old husband Derek
died from colorectal cancer in 2013

Cancer robbed us of our life and our future. We weren't intimate anymore and hadn't been the last two to three years of our marriage. We tried to have children from the moment we got engaged. We both had problems, but Derek's radiation for colorectal cancer made him sterile. Further, everything was so rushed in the beginning that we didn't have time, didn't process that we should bank some sperm.

Regardless, I do not have a child of Derek's. I don't know if that is a good thing or a bad thing. I am still debating that topic in my head. After Derek ended up with the colostomy bag, I became more of a nurse than a wife, I think. I changed his bag, changed his urine bag, changed and checked his wound VAC, gave him meds, and spent countless hours watching him sleep to make sure he was still breathing. Don't get me wrong, I love Derek with all my heart and soul, it just took a big toll on me and our relationship. We didn't often talk about how much we loved each other, I affirmed how much Derek loved me through other people and how he acted around me. He showed love by the way he acted, he didn't often come up and kiss me or hold my hand.

*

SUE NOVA
Sue's husband Dana died from
lung cancer in 2012 at age 46

I want to say that it brought us closer. We used to say that cancer was the worst best thing that ever happened to us. When he was still well enough, we were able to travel, eat, drink and be merry because we understood, truly, that tomorrow wasn't guaranteed. We got more real and open with each other. We talked about things that normally wouldn't be a part of our conversation. Like, do you want to be buried with shoes on or be in your favorite flip flops?

The only time, I believe, we ever parted ways on treatment was when there were no more viable treatment options and he wanted to find one. I looked this man, who I love, in the eye and told him it was okay if he didn't do any more. Part of me thinks he was relieved I said that. He asked me if I was sure. I said I was if he was. Then I made calls to make it happen.

*

SHERYL POCHEL
Sheryl's husband Brian died from
pancreatic cancer in 2011 at age 43

Brian and I were two different personality types. I was brought up in a family where mom and dad were best friends and worked together on everything. I never saw them fight, and I'm not sure that they ever did. Brian, on the other hand, was brought up by a mother who kept him from his father and treated him poorly. She wasn't physically abusive, and she loved him, but she just wasn't the kind of mother he deserved. I often say it was amazing that he turned out to be the man he was with her as his guide.

Given these different backgrounds, I was, and still am, a glass half full kind of person. Brian on the other hand was a "What glass?" type. While that might be a bit of an exaggeration, he was definitely the one who was more grounded in reality. This difference did cause problems in our relationship. I was often frustrated with his lack of willingness to try things that might help him feel better, or even survive.

We never really disagreed about his chemo treatments, I did a tremendous amount of research when it came to that. He trusted what I found. It was the extras we disagreed on. Mental health therapy, antidepressants and supplements, which was a big one for us. I felt like I was constantly pushing for him to make changes that would help improve his quality of life, and he always resisted those changes.

In the end, it was his body, his life, his decision. I will say that I still have a recurring dream where I'm begging him to take his supplements because if he doesn't, he will die.

*

KATHIE SCOTT
Kathie's 57-year-old husband Jim
died from prostate cancer in 2009

I think in most ways cancer made our marriage stronger. We were in the fight together and depended on each other to get through it. My husband often thanked me for taking care of him and I would remind him that, if the shoe were on the other foot, he would take care of me. Jim was a very easy patient, we just listened to the doctors and decided what needed to be done as far as treatments. The only time we had to convince him of anything was when we had to make a decision to go on a ventilator or not. My son-in-law was in the emergency room with me and promised him that he would make sure he would come off it if that became his choice down the road.

*

STEVE SHARP
Steve's 51-year-old wife Carolyn
died from melanoma in 2014

My relationship with Carolyn was greatly changed by her battle with cancer. Prior to her cancer diagnosis, she was very independent, working full time as a high school chemistry teacher, having both a bachelors and a master's degrees in chemistry. We tried every treatment offered in the hopes of beating the disease.

As her condition progressed, she became dependent on me. This caused stress in our relationship because her frustration caused her to be quick to anger with both myself and our youngest daughter. She often apologized, aware of what I would be going through after she passed away, since she had also lost a spouse. I found that to be very difficult to hear. Her condition was terminal, yet she was apologizing to me. It was so like my wife to put others first.

For the most part, we agreed with her course of treatment. Although when I was told that she only had two weeks to live, I shared the recommendation that she begin hospice and cease further treatment. Carolyn was a tremendous fighter and she didn't like the thought of quitting. When we discussed it, she agreed that it was time to stop treatment. I'll never forget the resigned look on her face as she finally realized that her days were numbered.

*

DIANNE WEST
Dianne's husband Vern died from
multiple myeloma in 2010 at age 69

Vern and I were best friends throughout our marriage. We could talk about anything and everything. When cancer entered our lives it drew us even closer. He relied heavily on me emotionally and physically. His medical team often remarked about what a strong team we were and how devoted I was to his care. Did I make mistakes? Of course I did. They are quite obvious when I re-read my Caring Bridge journal posts. But I must give myself a grace card because I know I was doing the best I could.

I believe that Vern was ready to stop fighting long before I was, but I didn't recognize it for some time. He would say he was tired or that he didn't want to do dialysis and I just did my positive talk and convinced him to keep on keeping on. I regret that I didn't hear what I now believe he was trying to tell me a few months before he died. We could have talked about it, weighed the options, figured out what the final straw might be, and agree how we would handle it.

*

A hero is an ordinary individual who finds
strength to persevere and endure
in spite of overwhelming obstacles.

CHRISTOPHER REEVE
*

CHAPTER TWELVE

Overwhelming Moments

Tenacity is not about avoiding being
overwhelmed but being indomitable in
the face of the overwhelming odds.
-ANDY DUNN

The needs of an ill loved one are at times overwhelming and stressful, which can lower our emotional threshold for feeling upset, put-upon, abandoned, and criticized. Feelings that get ignored can build like a volcano looking to vent steam. Did you ever experience moments of feeling overwhelmed, burdened, or resentful by your loved one's needs? How did you cope?

*

JANICE DEL VECCHIO
Janice lost her husband Stephen to bile duct cancer in 2006 at age 47,
and her second husband John to pancreatic cancer in 2013 at age 55

Absolutely. I think it is quite natural to feel this way. I had moments when I thought I wouldn't be able to handle all the emotions and exhaustion that went along with being the primary caregiver. I try to make time for myself when I could. I would talk to a friend or go out to dinner or lunch with friends. We tried to live as normal of a life as we could. I would try to keep busy and not just sit on the couch and feel sorry for myself.

There were times when both my husbands would get overly emotional and lash out at me. I would walk away and put some space between us. When it was calmer we would discuss what happened and would work it out. I also sought out counseling and it was the best thing I could have done for myself. Both hospitals that my husbands were treated at, also provided support for spouses. I was fortunate in that both were teaching hospitals in Boston and there were lots of resources available. Massage, yoga, etc.

*

CYNTHIA HORACEK
Cynthia's husband Don died from
rectal cancer in 2010 at age 57

I became stressed at times, of course. Who wouldn't? I think that having to help him with the ostomy started to cause some resentment on my part because I wanted him to be able to take care of it himself, and not wait for me to come home to help him change it. But I didn't really mind; I loved him so I would help him. I'd just take a deep breath and remind myself that I was glad he was still with me.

I had my mother to talk to, and also a wonderful therapist who really helped me get though his illness and the loss when he died.

*

MARGARET HUTSELL
Margaret's 77-year-old husband Tom
died from pancreatic cancer in 2016

Never burdened, never resentful, but overwhelmed, you bet. The hospital stays when we met with so many different doctors and staff we could never keep it all straight. The questions we would write down to ask and find out the doctors who could answer them would be in and out of Tom's room quicker than an eye blink!

The ongoing chemo treatments that were always given after labs were taken, lab results given, talking with the nurse, then the doctor and finally the chemo infusion lab. The forty-five-minute drive one way to and from the office, often twice a week if he needed saline to stay hydrated. It was our life, and we made it as good as we possibly could. Funny how I missed it after he died!

*

LYNN JORDAAN
Lynn's 58-year-old husband Johan
died from esophageal cancer in 2014

I did feel overwhelmed, I felt unqualified, but then who wouldn't. There was more anger and grief about the fact that this story, our story, wasn't going be the quintessential happy ending with two little old people walking off into the sunset holding hands. But no, I didn't feel resentful or burdened by his needs.

*

GAIL MARCHESA
Gail's husband John died from
colon cancer in 2009 at age 55

Yes, to all the emotions of overwhelmed and burdened. I think we all felt that one, but if you don't lash out it's all good.

*

HEATHER MCLAUGHLIN
Heather's 35-year-old husband Derek
died from colorectal cancer in 2013

I remember daily conversations with Dave, one of my assistant principals, who was also a good friend. He would let me just vent, cry, and try and work things through my head in his office. He would sit there and listen and try to be a voice of reason for me, but sometimes he would just be a sounding board. I can look back now and know that without that, I would have had a lot more breakdowns than I did. I felt overwhelmed when trying to juggle Derek's meds, what we called blowouts from his ostomy bag, and countless other medical stuff on top of all I had to do with teaching.

*

SUE NOVA
Sue's husband Dana died from
lung cancer in 2012 at age 46

I wasn't really overwhelmed in the beginning. We were around family a lot. I did keep the happy face on. No one really knew how treatment was going. He didn't want to worry his family, or mine. The kids, who were grown, knew what we told them. I was emotionally exhausted because of the facade I had to put on. Later, as he got sicker, I was exhausted emotionally and physically. That didn't matter though. There was no one he or I trusted to care for him. That was how it was until two weeks before he died. My daughter called hospice and told them that they needed to come help around the clock because I couldn't do it anymore.

*

SHERYL POCHEL
Sheryl's husband Brian died from
pancreatic cancer in 2011 at age 43

I often felt overwhelmed by our situation. Having a husband with cancer is something that I never want to experience EVER again. I took care of him, I took care of our kids, I managed his clinic. It was a lot. I wouldn't change a thing though. I did what I needed to do. I never felt burdened or resentful. I often felt tired. I took care of everyone else before myself. It has taken years for me to become the person I am now. His cancer and death shaped me into who I am today, and today I'm happy.

*

KATHIE SCOTT
Kathie's 57-year-old husband Jim
died from prostate cancer in 2009

I often felt overwhelmed but never burdened or resentful. His needs came first no matter what and it was my job and privilege to take care of him. Only one time did I flare up and give him a piece of my mind for not following doctor's orders. I don't regret it because I had met my breaking point and it needed to come out. I look at photos of myself taken toward the end and shortly afterward and I look just worn out but I would not go back and do anything differently.

*

STEVE SHARP
Steve's 51-year-old wife Carolyn
died from melanoma in 2014

I felt very guilty and angry that I would be the survivor and wondered why she was the one fighting a terminal illness. After all, she was six years younger. Both her grandmothers lived to age ninety-nine, and both her grandfathers lived into their late eighties.

After I made peace with God, I eventually came to realize that I had children to live for and it was not his will that I should die. He wanted me to make the most of every day, realize each day is a gift, and to be grateful that I was blessed to be married to such a wonderful woman. It took a lot of prayer and meditation for me to work through the negative emotions to discover feelings of gratitude.

*

DIANNE WEST
Dianne's husband Vern died from
multiple myeloma in 2010 at age 69

These were hard years, make no mistake. I didn't sleep well and didn't eat healthy. I actually do not know how I survived those years without becoming ill or injured myself. I'm five-foot-three, he was six feet tall, and having to lift him was difficult. But I learned how to do it safely and I prided myself on all of the things I was able to do. Most of his doctors assumed I was a nurse and were surprised that I had no background in that. I just loved my husband and wanted to do everything I possibly could to make him comfortable. And he was more comfortable when I was the one taking his blood pressure, hanging his IV meds, cleaning and changing his PICC line. His trust in the medical community had been damaged along the way. He trusted me. So when I was able to do these things, even just having me there in the room when others were doing these things, it made a huge difference for him.

There were moments I felt overwhelmed, but never burdened or resentful of the amount of care Vern required. Early on, when he finally came home after the diagnosis, surgeries and rehab, he was unkind to me during a visit with the home healthcare supervisor. This was very much unlike him, but he hurt my feelings nonetheless. Kathy, the nurse supervisor, noticed when I turned and stepped away silently. She finished talking to Vern and then came to me and gave me some wonderful advice. She said that Vern had been through so very much and he was scared and angry and needed to lash out. And he could only do that to someone he knew loved him unconditionally and would never leave him. I believed that and knew it to be true. And I held onto those words whenever they were needed.

*

Taking care of yourself physically
can improve your mental health.

DR. ERLANGER A. TURNER
*

CHAPTER THIRTEEN

Our Own Health

Health is a state of complete physical, mental, and
social well-being. -WORLD HEALTH ORGANIZATION

As our anatomical and physiological systems work in tandem with our emotional well-being, when one part of our body is stressed, other parts become compromised. How did the stress of your loved one's cancer affect your own health?

*

JANICE DEL VECCHIO
Janice lost her husband Stephen to bile duct cancer in 2006 at age 47,
and her second husband John to pancreatic cancer in 2013 at age 55

It took a toll on me. I gained weight and stopped working out. I sought help for stress and depression. I kept most of my appointments I had for my own medical issues. I was diagnosed with breast cancer about three months before I married my second husband. I completed treatment but still had to go to several follow up appointments. During both of my experiences with losing a spouse, I had to postpone planned surgeries. The first involved a torn meniscus in my left knee and the second time was a left hip replacement. I waited until both had passed away before having surgery.

*

CYNTHIA HORACEK
Cynthia's husband Don died from
rectal cancer in 2010 at age 57

I can't really say that the stress of Don's cancer affected my own health. I knew I had to stay strong for him, and on some level, that meant my own health had to stay good. It was during the final few days when Don was dying that I started losing it more and more, but I never let him see me cry. That was when I didn't eat much, and I didn't even want to go to the bathroom for fear of missing his last moments. I would never have forgiven myself if I wasn't there when he took his last breath. I don't know why that was so important to me, but it was.

I know a lot of people who are dying will actually wait until their loved one isn't with them to die because they don't want their loved one to go through that. But I'm glad I was there to hold his hand. I told him I loved him, and that it was okay for him to go. I wanted to tell him not to leave me, but knew I had to give him permission to die. I wanted to make his transition as easy for him as possible.

*

MARGARET HUTSELL
Margaret's 77-year-old husband Tom
died from pancreatic cancer in 2016

It didn't seem to affect me a lot. My annual physical was put aside the year he was sick, but within two months following his death, I made my appointment and came away with a clean bill of health. I love to sleep and would nap every time Tom would nap. The laundry and cleaning could wait.

Following his passing, my sleep habits became erratic and still give me fits some nights. As I write this post, it has been over a year since Tom transitioned to his next reality. I am sad and lonely, and feel as though I have no idea who I am now. I know I need to find new friends who understand what I feel. Now that I am alone for the first time in my life at age seventy-eight, I need to dig deep for strength to find joy again.

*

LYNN JORDAAN
Lynn's 58-year-old husband Johan
died from esophageal cancer in 2014

I felt more anxiety over what would happen when he was gone, and so went off to the family doctor who prescribed antidepressants. Eating was a problem, but only because I don't enjoy eating alone, and due to the nature of his cancer, Johan wasn't eating much right from the beginning. I was lucky in that I worked with a company who was very supportive and while I was at work, my bosses and coworkers ensure that at least during the week, someone would have lunch with me, so I was eating at least eating one meal a day. I was also seeing a social worker who was attached to the facility where Johan was getting chemo, and therefore was experienced in anticipatory grief and all that comes with that. I was able to scream and shout and let go of what was bothering my psyche twice per week.

I also joined a peer support group with the Cancer Cares Society in Canada and spoke to a volunteer there once or twice a week.

*

GAIL MARCHESA
Gail's husband John died from
colon cancer in 2009 at age 55

It was after John's death when I had more anxiety than usual, and took some meds. Being alone and in charge was a bit scary.

*

HEATHER MCLAUGHLIN
Heather's 35-year-old husband Derek
died from colorectal cancer in 2013

I had severe migraines. I had very sore muscles. I was not very hungry, so I didn't eat much. I found out later that I was keeping everything bottled up inside, which isn't good and with everything that we went through, was diagnosed with PTSD. I don't suffer from all the effects of PTSD any more, but the wail of a fire truck or the sirens of an ambulance on the east coast does give me slight anxiety. I still have migraines. I still have very sore muscles in my neck and back and will most likely always have that. I am always tired. Partly because I am a teacher, partly because I miss Derek so much I think some part of me will always be a little depressed. As a widow, I have an odd sense of humor, but if something gets under my skin, I can't take it. I had to put my dog, Rio, down in July and couldn't stay in the room with Rio for very long after he was dead. Don't know why, just couldn't. I had to grieve someplace else. I have my ups and downs. They can range from week to week, day-to-day, minute to minute. It can depend on the trigger; and I still get triggers that I am unaware of.

*

SUE NOVA
Sue's husband Dana died from
lung cancer in 2012 at age 46

Aside from the exhaustion, I ate all my feelings. I couldn't drink because I never knew what the night would bring. So I ate. I ate my way to about three hundred pounds. I tried to exercise regularly, however that was difficult. So I ate.

*

SHERYL POCHEL
Sheryl's husband Brian died from
pancreatic cancer in 2011 at age 43

Brian's cancer did affect my health. I remember the day he went in for his preop exam, the one that was going to tell us what kind of cancer he had. I broke down crying uncontrollably on my bedroom floor. It was at that moment when I knew I needed help and couldn't do this on my own. I called my doctor's office and they got me in that day for an appointment for antidepressants. I'm glad I did that. It helped to keep me more even keel throughout the years. I also talked with the cancer psychologist at the hospital on a regular basis. He was a pillar of strength for me.

Unfortunately my weight also took a turn for the worse. Over the course of those years I gained over forty pounds. I am four-foot-ten and one hundred eighty-four pounds; that's not a good weight for me. I started losing some in the last months of Brian's life because of all of the running I was doing, and I lost more after he died. People would ask me "What are you doing to lose weight?" My response was, "I went on the My Husband Died and I Can't Eat and Throw Up When I Do diet, I don't recommend it." That weight stayed off for a couple of years, but slowly crept back up again because of some very stressful situations. In the last year I have put myself first and I have worked to lost the weight again. I have lost seventy-five pounds and I feel better than I have in years. I'm better at putting myself first now and making my needs a priority.

*

KATHIE SCOTT
Kathie's 57-year-old husband Jim
died from prostate cancer in 2009

I didn't suffer any health issues during that time. I consider myself to be very strong physically and mentally. I was blessed to stay healthy. I had some anxiety issues and problems sleeping after Jim passed away but was able to work through them with a little help from my doctor.

*

STEVE SHARP
Steve's 51-year-old wife Carolyn
died from melanoma in 2014

The high level of stress dealing with Carolyn's diagnosis was very difficult for me to handle. I couldn't sleep, was exhausted, and lost weight due to a lack of hunger. I remember feeling very inadequate. As her husband, I wanted to protect my wife but protecting her from cancer was beyond my control. I thought I was a failure. My physician prescribed medication to deal with anxiety. It also allowed me to sleep enough to barely function.

I knew my wife was terminal and anticipated her death. It was as though she was restrained to the ties of a railroad track with a freight train bearing down on her. My sad thoughts prevented me from living fully in the present and I spent too much time worrying about the future. I was blessed by family and friends who made sure that I was eating something and getting rest.

*

DIANNE WEST
Dianne's husband Vern died from
multiple myeloma in 2010 at age 69

I was very lucky to remain healthy during my husband's cancer years. I somehow existed on three to four hours of sleep during the week as I juggled work with Vern's dialysis, doctor appointments, and chemo treatments. But then on the weekends I would nap when Vern napped to catch up.

He spent the first twelve weeks in hospitals and rehabs. Some allowed me to stay with him overnight, some did not. He did better when I was there, so I spent a lot of time in those facilities with him. I had a little rolling bag with my laptop and work projects, a change of clothes and personal items so I could stay whenever possible.

I cannot recommend that others do what I did, but it was what I needed and wanted to do. I let other things go so I could do what was needed for him. During that first year he was pretty much confined to bed, with short times doing physical therapy. We had a hospital bed set up in the living room and he had a Foley catheter and a colostomy (that was done about six months after diagnosis). I kept that room squeaky clean but I let the rest of the house go.

I did not take good care of myself. I really didn't even think about it. People would suggest I get a massage, go to a spa; they'd even give me a gift card. I never used them. I could not imagine leaving him to do something for myself. I know that is ridiculous and unhealthy, but it is how I felt. I have a very strong faith and belief in God and was assured that I was doing what I was supposed to be doing and I would be okay.

*

CHAPTER FOURTEEN

Juggling Our Emotions

Heavy hearts, like heavy clouds, are best
relieved by the letting go of a little water.
-ANTOINE RIVAROL

Cancer forces us into an emotional juggling act between anticipatory grief, fear, isolation, determination, and hope—and tests our ability to precariously balance all these emotions sometimes in a single moment. While caring for your loved one, what emotions were hardest for you to juggle?

*

JANICE DEL VECCHIO
Janice lost her husband Stephen to bile duct cancer in 2006 at age 47,
and her second husband John to pancreatic cancer in 2013 at age 55

Anticipatory grief and fear. I was open about the amount of sadness that I felt and that I didn't want to lose them. I managed to keep to myself that I was already grieving their loss before they passed on. I thought it was best to not share that with either as they were both worried about themselves and what would their deaths would do to me. I definitely sought out help for this. I worked with a social worker at both hospitals that were trained in grief and caregiving. It was a tremendous relief to have someone who understood the emotions that I was feeling.

*

CYNTHIA HORACEK
Cynthia's husband Don died from
rectal cancer in 2010 at age 57

The hardest emotion for me to juggle was my fear. I had no idea how to go on without my husband. He was my everything—my partner, my best friend, my advisor, my support, and my purpose. I couldn't imagine my life without him. That and also trying to be positive for him and our daughters. That was hard. I kept up a brave front and never let him see me cry, when all I wanted to do was have him hold me while I cried.

*

MARGARET HUTSELL
Margaret's 77-year-old husband Tom
died from pancreatic cancer in 2016

I had trouble with fear of the future, of death itself, of loneliness, of purpose, and whether I could even live without Tom. After we had been married for fifty-seven years, it seemed almost impossible to go on without him by my side. My friends drifted away into their own lives, which we expected. Our family and the few friends who remained connected wanted time with their dad, grandpa, friend. And I? Well, I wanted all of him. I did not want to share him (well, maybe with family), but realized there would never be enough time together and I became the woman I never wanted to be.

I found an awesome therapist through one of the dear nurses who helped us understand what was going on and who was there each and every time we needed support. Tom didn't begin therapy with me, but after coming along one time, he never stayed home after that. We both received unbelievable support and loving care from Sandi, and five days before Tom died, he asked her to please continue to help me as I wandered through the maze and fog of grief.

*

LYNN JORDAAN
Lynn's 58-year-old husband Johan
died from esophageal cancer in 2014

I think the overriding emotion was sadness, and then anger. Sadness to see this amazing robust man slowly become more and more wracked in pain and feeling powerless to make it better for him, then anger at that powerlessness and anger that our story was ending. We were supposed to end our lives together after many years of sitting on the porch in our rocking chairs together. Anger that someone this strong could be caught off guard by cancer. He was supposed to be my protector, how could he do this when he wasn't here to catch me if and when I fell.

I did see a psychologist while Johan was ill, she explained that this was anticipatory guilt. It was helpful to have a name put to the jumble of feelings I was experiencing. However, it didn't help to realize I was grieving before he had even died. Did this mean I was wishing him dead? That I had given up on him? I did not like this at all. It did help to know that this was a normal situation and that others felt this way too. I wasn't some kind of monster, who didn't care enough, who just wanted to get to the end of this already.

*

GAIL MARCHESA
Gail's husband John died from
colon cancer in 2009 at age 55

I would sit and think I would want to go. He would sign me up, so I thought it couldn't hurt. How was I going to do everything by myself? I bounced between, "Hey, I can do this," and then bounced right back to I can't.

I kept in touch with the chaplain from hospice and he told me about a group that meets for a ten-week period. I thought I would try. It turned out to be hard in the first two weeks, but after that it was good for me. I learned a lot of things, like I wasn't crazy, everyone goes through it. In the course of a year, I brought one of my friends after her husband passed and we made many friends. I moved from South Carolina to New Jersey, and we still keep in touch. I also started volunteering with hospice, doing condolence cards and such. It kind of made me feel close to John.

*

HEATHER MCLAUGHLIN
Heather's 35-year-old husband Derek
died from colorectal cancer in 2013

The hardest emotions to juggle were thoughts of the future. I can remember Derek saying things like, "When I am gone...," and "When you get married again..." Those were very difficult for me to hear because I never wanted to accept that Derek would actually die. I thought some miracle drug would come out or somehow his body would figure out how to fight off the cancer.

Another emotion that was really hard was the overwhelming feelings and depression of it all. When I finally sat down and thought of my life at the current time, I couldn't believe everything I was going through and that we were actually doing it. It made me very tired to think of everything we were doing to try to fight the cancer, which never actually worked.

*

SUE NOVA
Sue's husband Dana died from
lung cancer in 2012 at age 46

In the beginning, I thought Dana wasn't trying hard enough to not feel sick. Meaning, basically, I thought he needed to man up and act not sick. So I was angry. I was angry, too, because our whole damn life had been turned upside down and sideways. I didn't blame him; I knew this wasn't his fault. I just was angry. In retrospect, I suppose I was grieving the life we were losing. I also knew that no matter how the journey ended, I would lose the only man I ever loved.

I didn't seek any outside help. I always have been pretty good at working out my feelings on my own. Logic will override my emotions and I can see things more clear. Is that for everyone? I don't know. All I know is that it worked for me.

*

SHERYL POCHEL
Sheryl's husband Brian died from
pancreatic cancer in 2011 at age 43

Being so young when Brian was diagnosed with a death sentence was the hardest thing I ever had to go through. Everything was so jumbled in the beginning. It was impossible to comprehend that my husband, the father of my kids, could die. Every once in a while I would let the fact that he could die creep in, which was painful and brought me to instant tears, though years later that pain seemed like nothing compared to the real thing. The idea of being an only parent was terrifying. How was I supposed to do this all by myself? How was I supposed to raise these four beautiful kids all alone? I think that was the hardest thing, knowing that my kids hearts would be broken and there was nothing I could do to make that better.

I wear my emotions on my sleeve. I can't hide much nor hold it in. I have no problem telling people how I feel. I did see the cancer psychologist and also talked with the social worker at the hospital to help me deal with Brian's cancer. I also talked to my close friends and family about what was going on and what I was feeling. I feel like when I needed something emotionally I was willing to get the help I needed.

*

KATHIE SCOTT
Kathie's 57-year-old husband Jim
died from prostate cancer in 2009

I will admit that many of my emotions during the more than five years of care giving were held inside of me. While I shared some of them with a couple of close friends, I could never let myself completely go and admit how mad and how scared I was for the future. My mind kept telling me to keep the good, positive face on and don't give in to the inevitable. I felt if I admitted the complete and honest truth to myself that I was giving up hope and that would be our downfall. I took my anger and fear out on my pillow, my steering wheel, the phone, or whatever else I could slam or beat up on in seclusion. In the beginning, my boss, who had been through cancer treatment himself, took me in his arms and let me cry and told me whatever I needed would be made available. I never sought any professional help or support because, once again, that was admitting defeat and the loss of hope and I simply could not do it. When the test results were not positive, I would put the happy face and positive attitude on and get through it. In retrospect, I'm not sure this was good for any of us.

*

STEVE SHARP
Steve's 51-year-old wife Carolyn
died from melanoma in 2014

I had to deal with so many difficult emotions while caring for my wife Carolyn. The hardest emotions for me to cope with were anger and guilt.

I was so angry because I couldn't believe that I was going to be a widower again. I had been through this just fifteen years before. Certainly I had experienced more than my share of loss and grief!

I also felt very guilty. My wife was a far better person than I. She had dedicated her life to teaching young people. My wife touched so many students. Long after her passing, I was approached by her former students who let me know what a positive impact that she had had on their lives. Although her life was cut short, it had a lot of depth and meaning. How is it fair that such a selfless person would live such a short life?

It wasn't easy for me to be open with my emotions. Yet, I was blessed to have family and friends who I could talk to about my feelings. I don't know how I would have coped without having these people listen to me.

*

DIANNE WEST
Dianne's husband Vern died from
multiple myeloma in 2010 at age 69

I kept my emotions pretty much to myself while caring for Vern, and that's something I would not necessarily recommend to others. It was important for me to be stoic for my husband. He was going through so much that I needed to be strong for him, to make sure he believed that we'd get through every crisis that hit us. If I felt tears were close to the surface, I would just step into another room out of his eyesight to gain my composure.

I don't think any of my friends ever saw my deep racking sobs. Those happened at home, in the shower, in the car, when I was alone. I've generally been that way most of my life. I deflect when someone asks how I am doing by immediately asking them a question about themselves. It works every time. But this behavior also gave others the impression that I was doing quite well and didn't need support of any kind. And that was not true.

There honestly was no time for me to seek professional support for myself, especially those last two years. And I don't think that would have helped me handle those years any better than I did without it. Working, caring for Vern and staying on top of the household duties took up all of my waking hours. But since I wasn't sleeping well, my night hours could often be spent online where I found the Association of Cancer Online Resources (www.acor.org). This was a safe outlet for me to express my fears and concerns with other caregivers and patients who were dealing with multiple myeloma. I could ask questions and someone else was bound to have experienced the same thing and would share what had worked for them. That online community helped me greatly and I actually met several of these wonderful people in person years later within the widowed community.

*

Consult not your fears but your
hopes and your dreams.

POPE JOHN XXIII
*

CHAPTER FIFTEEN

Facing Our Fears

The oldest and strongest emotion of mankind is
fear, and the oldest and strongest kind of fear
is fear of the unknown. -H. P. LOVECRAFT

The fear of death has been hardwired into us all. And yet cancer is synonymous with death. For some, having a deadline offers a chance to sort things into order. For others, it induces paralyzing anxiety. At what point did you and your loved one reconcile with the probability of death as the only outcome?

*

JANICE DEL VECCHIO
Janice lost her husband Stephen to bile duct cancer in 2006 at age 47,
and her second husband John to pancreatic cancer in 2013 at age 55

I felt that both husbands and their medical teams did everything that was possible to treat their cancers and prolong the quality of life for both. Both husbands died of similar cancers; bile duct and pancreatic cancers. Both have no cure. We were fortunate that we were in an area with some of the best hospitals in the world and we had great medical coverage. It was heartbreaking hoping that the various drug trials would work. There would be some positive results but more often than not it was not the case. A doctor told me once that not knowing is actually worse than knowing. It further explained that once you know, good or bad, a plan can then be made. I found this to be fairly accurate. I experienced such a wide range of emotions during both illnesses. Hope, desperation, fear, anxiety, helplessness, dread, heartbreak are the most memorable. Both husbands didn't find out they were dying and that no further treatment was available when they were both about two weeks from dying. That is how we wanted it. We didn't want a time frame until all treatment possibilities were exhausted. I wouldn't change that even if I have the unfortunate experience of having to go through it a third time.

*

CYNTHIA HORACEK
Cynthia's husband Don died from
rectal cancer in 2010 at age 57

We didn't deal with the probability of death until the very end, when we found out the cancer had metastasized, and the doctor told us he had several days to a few weeks left. When he was first diagnosed, I told him, "You're not allowed to die." But that didn't work out very well. Calling my daughter to come home from across the country "now" was hard. She was walking home from school when I called her. I asked if her boyfriend was home. He was, but she wasn't. I told her to call me when she got home, but she said, "No, tell me now," and I did.

I still feel my husband got the best care he could have had, and I definitely never felt his doctors gave up on him. Don had a positive attitude throughout the entire ordeal of having cancer. He never felt sorry for himself or got into self-pity or gave up. His body was just too weak to fight anymore.

*

MARGARET HUTSELL
Margaret's 77-year-old husband Tom
died from pancreatic cancer in 2016

It was only after Tom experienced seventeen rounds of weekly chemo treatments with the second oncologist. His CAT showed what was expected to be cancer growth in his peritoneum and we knew immediately that this was not good. Tom asked about clinical trials, but because of his metastasis and the type of cancer (pancreatic) there were none available to him. The doctor suggested it might be time to live without any further treatment or interference in our daily lives and consider hospice care at home. We were expecting this sooner or later, and sooner became reality. We were numb.

As we left the oncology clinic, nurses lined up with sad faces and some had tears running down their cheeks. Tom was a favored patient because he was so pleasant to work with and for. We were sad and frightened but resolved to live each day to the absolute fullest extent. We actually planned a five-day trip to Las Vegas with our children and their spouses. Tom loved every single minute of the trip, refusing to use the wheelchair provided by hospice. Two weeks after returning home, he transitioned into the next reality.

*

LYNN JORDAAN
Lynn's 58-year-old husband Johan
died from esophageal cancer in 2014

I'm not sure when Johan came to the realization he was dying, but I had a few markers, if you will. One was watching him dance with my daughter at her wedding. I realized this was probably the last time he would dance with her, with me, or anyone else ever again. He did everything he could to make that day special and memorable for her. It was as if he knew it would soon be downhill.

The next marker came on Christmas Eve 2013, when his sister from Zimbabwe paid us a surprise visit. Watching him hold on to her for dear life, I knew then we wouldn't have much longer. It was like a switch turning off. When he said goodbye to her at the airport, the next switch went off. After that farewell, he asked that no one come and visit anymore, he wanted to have his friends and family remember him as he was. Do I feel he gave up? In a way, yes, he did. He was ready to go, and told me so before the diagnosis was even made. This made it even harder to accept when the time came.

*

GAIL MARCHESA
Gail's husband John died from
colon cancer in 2009 at age 55

I believe John and his doctor decided he was done with chemo in January, but John never told me. Somehow I only really believed he was done when he went on hospice. I think that's called denial.

*

HEATHER MCLAUGHLIN
Heather's 35-year-old husband Derek
died from colorectal cancer in 2013

I think Derek reconciled with death long before I did. We learned that the cancer was terminal, or metastatic, in August 2012, from the doctors. We knew it was terminal the moment he had his heart attack in May 2012. I think this is when Derek realized and reconciled with it. I was still hoping for a miracle.

I can't honestly tell you when I reconciled with the thought of losing Derek. It might have been Thanksgiving 2012, when the school put me on FMLA and told me to go spend time with Derek before he died. It might have been after the EMS banquet dinner in December 2012, when Derek was awarded the lifetime member award and there was this amazing speech given about him. Unfortunately, he felt so bad he couldn't go, but I went in his place and accepted his awarded on his behalf.

I don't really know if it wasn't until about twenty-four to thirty-six hours before his passing when he asked me to have his boss turn off his work phone (he was that dedicated), or when we were moving his almost lifeless body to the ambulance for the ride to the hospice house where he would spend the last nineteen hours of his life.

I think at each of these times, more of me realized and partially reconciled with Derek's dying, although nothing, I mean nothing, prepares you for that.

*

SUE NOVA
Sue's husband Dana died from
lung cancer in 2012 at age 46

I don't think he ever did. I will rephrase that. If he did, he never said so to me. I know he had private conversations with his Spiritual Father, and I believe they spoke about it. I know him and I think that's not something he would have wanted to put on me, regardless of what the obvious was. Just to get him to finally quit chemo, he asked me if I was sure. He probably would have continued until the wheels fell off.

*

SHERYL POCHEL
Sheryl's husband Brian died from
pancreatic cancer in 2011 at age 43

The idea of Brian actually dying seemed impossible. When he was diagnosed he was given "a year, probably not two," and told he would never be a candidate for surgery to remove his tumor.

He did everything he was told to do. Radiation. Chemotherapy. Medications galore. Then one day a woman showed up at our house. She had with her a nutritional supplement. She said she felt awkward being there, but that she was compelled to be. She handed me the supplement and told me to have Brian take it, that she had personally known people who had survived cancers by using this and she wanted him to try it. He did and things started to change. He felt better. He had more energy. Chemo didn't have as negative of an effect on him.

Then, eight months after being diagnosed, his tumor stopped shrinking. We were sure that we were at the beginning of the end. Then his oncologist said something that we never expected him to say "I think we should talk with the surgeon and see if she can take your tumor out." Fast forward, he had the surgery called a Whipple. It is a massive surgery that removes part of the pancreas, gallbladder, bile duct, part of the stomach and some small intestine. It took over eight hours to do.

The surgeon sent the pathology to the lab as she removed bits and pieces, and nothing came back as cancerous. Three days later the final pathology was in and there was no cancer. None. This was the first time at the UW Hospital that this had ever happened. It was amazing. I wholeheartedly believe that this was a result of the supplement that Brian was taking. However, it was expensive and our income was limited so Brian quit taking it. I begged him not to, but he didn't feel he could justify the money. Fifteen months later, he had a recurrence in his lung and another tumor in his brain. No matter what I said he wouldn't take the supplement again.

He had surgery and whole brain radiation for the brain tumor and we waited for a while to start the chemo again. I again begged him to restart the supplements. He wouldn't. This is one of the hardest things for me. I was mad at him for not trying. I was mad that he was so stubborn. Five and a half years later, I still have a recurring dream about it. In my dream he's alive (though I can't tell if he's still alive or was dead and came back to life), and I'm begging him to take his supplements. I keep telling him that if he doesn't, I know he will die (because even in my dreams I know that he is still dead). But he still won't take them. I believe they helped him live as long as he did, and I believe that he may still be here if he hadn't quit. It is painful to have that unfounded belief, but it is there. I can't help it.

*

KATHIE SCOTT
Kathie's 57-year-old husband Jim
died from prostate cancer in 2009

My husband never gave up until his last ten days on earth. He was a fighter and did everything he could and anything the doctors suggested to make more time. There was no discussion about quality versus quantity in our household. About ten days prior to his death, he began having mild strokes and everything rapidly failed. His doctor said she believed the strokes robbed him of the ability to understand he needed to fight.

During that last hospital stay Jim had an episode that brought everyone running, bed flattened in preparation for a code. He looked and me and said, "I'm out of here." Confused, I asked him what he was talking about. He gave me a look of "Don't you see what's happening?" I realized he knew the end was near.

After almost eight years my heart breaks, knowing that he was probably scared but never voiced it. I can hardly bear to think of it even now.

*

STEVE SHARP
Steve's 51-year-old wife Carolyn
died from melanoma in 2014

Even though Carolyn and I were told by a neurologist that she was terminal, we didn't accept his opinion because her oncologist gave her a life expectancy of two more years which we wanted to believe. Carolyn tried every possible treatment to fight her cancer. We both were optimists and believed that if she was still alive there was a chance to survive.

It wasn't until her last MRI showed that none of treatments had stopped the growth of the cancer in her brain, that we were forced to accept the truth: she only had two weeks to live. This news hit me like a ton of bricks. At this point, Carolyn entered hospice care and although we wanted to get her home, the pain from tumors was not manageable at home. Perhaps, if I been realistic rather than overly optimistic, Carolyn could have spent her remaining time at home. As a result, I felt that I had let Carolyn down and felt deep regret.

*

DIANNE WEST
Dianne's husband Vern died from
multiple myeloma in 2010 at age 69

Vern's infectious disease doctor was a no-nonsense guy who we both liked. He told it like it was, but with compassion. He shared early on that he hoped they could give Vern eighteen months, although he said he believed an infection, not the cancer, would be what took Vern's life. We knew there was no cure for multiple myeloma, but also knew some lived longer than expected. When he passed that eighteen-month mark and was in partial remission, we thought we were going to be one of the lucky ones.

The doctor who did Vern's abdominal aortic pseudoaneurysm surgery was an excellent surgeon but had a huge God complex. He made the statement that Vern was going to die. This was about a year before his death. Vern was devastated. It dashed the hope I had worked so hard to keep alive. On our way home from that appointment, we talked about it and I helped him switch his anger at the doctor for his insensitivity and not to focus on the actual words he said. It seemed to help although since Vern didn't speak about his feelings very often, he might have just been doing that for my benefit.

Other than that, we did not accept that death was imminent until the day we signed the papers for him to transfer to hospice. He was on dialysis. And when I asked the hospice nurse how we were going to manage his dialysis she gently explained that he would not be able to continue dialysis if he moved to hospice. That was a reality smack upside the head. I remember turning to Vern and asking him what he wanted to do and making sure he understood what this meant. His words were, "Why delay the inevitable?" as he signed the papers.

Vern had fought so very hard and had experienced so many unexpected setbacks. When I look back at those last several months I can see his decline, but when I was living it, I did not. I believe that he hung on longer than he wanted because he knew I wasn't ready yet. I feel badly about that, but I honestly did not see the end was so near.

CHAPTER SIXTEEN

The Final Days

Moments are fleeting. Memories are permanent.
Love is forever. -LYNDA CHELDELIN FELL

Even when death is expected and your loved one's final days are coming to a close, it's common to feel myriad of emotions. When that final breath is drawn, some feel a sense of shock and disbelief while others feel relieved to know their loved one is no longer in pain. What were your loved one's final days, hours, and last moment like?

*

JANICE DEL VECCHIO
Janice lost her husband Stephen to bile duct cancer in 2006 at age 47, and her second husband John to pancreatic cancer in 2013 at age 55

My first husband went into liver failure about twenty-four hours before he died. He was still able to communicate but his body was violently shaking. I told him I loved him, and he said it back to me. He was worried about me but I couldn't make out everything he was saying. I reassured him I would be okay and he wasn't to worry. He calmed down quite a bit after that and then became nonresponsive.

His mother was there the day he died. Friends came by and asked me to go for dinner with them. I checked with the hospice nurse and she said that I should go. We went to a nearby restaurant. When I got back, Steve was breathing heavy and seemed agitated. He had a morphine pump and I was told I could press it to help calm him down. It worked and he seemed calmer.

His mother was unsure if she should stay or not. I told her it was up to her, and she decided to leave. I got undressed and got ready for bed. I had just laid down when the hospice nurse alerted me that Steve was actively dying. He passed away just before midnight on Friday, October 13. I laughed a little bit and explained to the nurse that my husband had a morbid fear of Friday the 13th. I couldn't believe the irony of the whole situation. Soon enough, the tears came. I was alone and called my sister to let her know that Steve had died and then called my mother-in-law. That was a very difficult call to make as she had decided to leave instead of staying. I really believe that Steve waited for me to get back from dinner and for us to be alone when he died.

For a while, I also wondered whether the dose of morphine I gave Steve caused him to die. I was assured he was actively dying and if anything I made it easier for him to leave.

We did not preplan the funeral arrangements. That was what we both wanted. We didn't want to deal with it until we had too. While I waited for my sister to meet me at the hospice facility, I called the funeral home we wanted to use and got that underway. I packed up my clothes and cleaned up the room. I also sprinkled Steve with holy water and said prayers for him. He had been given last rites earlier that day by our priest. I left shortly after my sister arrived and I went home.

John, my second husband, had a procedure at Massachusetts General Hospital to relieve fluid buildup in his stomach the day before he died. He came through it well and was still able to communicate. He told me he loved me, and I said it back. He eventually stopped talking but was able to squeeze my hand if I asked him a direct yes or no question.

I was asked if I wanted to move him to a hospice facility. I had the representative come and meet with me but decided I didn't want him to go through the trauma of being moved, and the hospital said he could stay until he passed away. He eventually went into a coma and his breathing became more labored. I stayed with him until 5 p.m. the day he died. I decided to get out of the room for a bit and went across the street to have dinner. Everyone knew where I was and had my contact info. His son and son-in-law were in the room with John. I came back about forty-five minutes later and both were still there. John wasn't crazy about his son-in-law and I wasn't either. I went right over to John and said that I was back and his agitated breathing became more steady. His son-in-law finally left. It was just me and his son Michael. About an hour later John started to code and I knew he was dying. He died with me holding him and telling him it was okay to leave. John fought it right to the end. I really feel he waited for me to come back to the room before he died. I think he wanted just me and his son with him.

Like the experience with my first husband, Steve, John and I did not want any preplanning done. We both wanted to wait until he passed to make the arrangements. I called and started the process. The hospital nurse came in and confirmed he was gone and was very supportive and kind to me and John's son. We made a few phone calls to let people know, and I started the process of removing personal effects. His son Mike and I lived at the hospital together for about two weeks. He came home when I told him that it was getting near the end of his dad's life. I will always be grateful to him for that. He was a great comfort to both me and John.

*

CYNTHIA HORACEK
Cynthia's husband Don died from
rectal cancer in 2010 at age 57

The end was fast which was a blessing for my husband. He had a bone marrow biopsy on Friday, came home Saturday, we got the prognosis on Tuesday, and he died on Friday.

I wasn't happy with the hospice we had, and I had heard such wonderful things about other hospice care. I had to practically beg the hospice doctor for morphine and had been promised that Don wouldn't suffer, but he did. The doctor said, "If he's on morphine he won't be able to communicate with you," which first of all, isn't true, but Don couldn't communicate anyway as he wasn't lucid for most of the time. Even a hour of suffering was too long as far as I was concerned.

I sat by his bed those last three days, telling him it was okay to go. I wanted to say, "Don't leave me," but it was all about him, not about me. Our daughters were also there, and my daughter's now-husband was there to support her, but he ended up supporting me, too. I was grateful for all of the support I had around me.

On the last morning, Don kept looking up at the ceiling and reaching up to something only he could see. I knew he wasn't hallucinating. Suddenly, he said, "Well, I guess so," as clear as a bell and took his last breath. I held his hand and laid my head on his chest. When he was gone, I climbed into the bed and held him. Our dog jumped up and laid his chin on Don's thigh and licked his hand. He stayed with me until the mortuary came to pick Don up. The dog wasn't allowed on the beds, but they say animals know.

One thing I feel bad about is that I don't know if I told him how much I loved him. I most likely did, when I told him how much we all loved him and how wonderful a husband and father he had been. But it still kind of haunts me at times. Did he know how much I loved him?

*

MARGARET HUTSELL
Margaret's 77-year-old husband Tom
died from pancreatic cancer in 2016

Three days before he died, Tom took our new SUV to the grocery store, all by himself (his request) and was outside puttering in his yard (his favorite place to be). He was pitifully thin and his muscle tone was gone, but he persevered in making every day special in some way. His appetite was good and he was able to sleep through the night. His ascites was slowing down and every other medical task we did daily was done without any problem.

Two days before he died, Tom seemed to lose his capacity to get up from a chair or the toilet seat without a lot of help. Hospice had provided a lovely new walker with large wheels and he finally started to use it and joked that he was training for a walker marathon. He continued to eat and drink without assistance and, although in smaller amounts, it was whatever he wanted to eat at the time. He moved about the house with ease, joked and talked normally, and his laughter was often and hearty.

The day before he died, he woke up and asked for strawberry pancakes and chocolate milk for breakfast, walked to the kitchen and sat and ate all his food. Our son and daughter-in-law came to stay with me two days prior. Since I had to have help getting Tom up from the toilet seat, they decided I shouldn't be alone. Both my husband and son sat at the table and ate together, talking about the Cubs World Series win, and enjoying themselves. Tom felt tired afterwards, and walked back to our bedroom and took a nap for about an hour.

After his nap, he came back out into the family room (again with his new shiny walker) and watched TV for a while. He seemed to tire easily and decided to get back on the bed and watch TV.

And then everything changed just like that. He was himself, eating, drinking, had a cold pear and a cherry Pepsi. All of a sudden, he became agitated, trying to lift himself up from the bed, rocking back and forth to do so, without success. He would answer questions by grunting. No more words. By 4 p.m., I called hospice and the nurse came along with the social worker. They told us "something had changed," and I should call our son in Chicago and he should plan on coming up within the next few days to see his dad before he died. As the early evening arrived, our daughter came from her teaching job and our son and daughter-in-law left for home, with the plan of returning in the morning to stay the course.

Tom continued to rock and started to moan softly and had to go to the bathroom. He could not get out of bed or speak words, just soft grunts when asked questions about his comfort or pain level. He continued to moan and move his arms around in the air, his legs up and down on the bed and, in general, was almost in constant motion.

I called for another hospice nurse and she got to the house around 10 p.m. She thought it was time to administer some morphine and Ativan just in case Tom was in pain and that was causing the agitation, since by that time he could not tell us in words. I gave him one dose of morphine and one dose of Ativan but nothing seemed to lessen the movement or moaning.

At about 4 a.m., my daughter and I decided to give Tom oxygen. That seemed to calm him and he stopped moaning and began to rest. He did not want covers on him, nor did he want a pillow under his head. His breathing slowed, as did his heartbeat. Without a sound, he took his last breath and left for heaven at 5 a.m. He died as he wanted— at home in his own bed with family by his side.

There is never enough time. We knew for fourteen months he was dying. We had a wonderfully special final year plus two months together. But after fifty-seven years, the shock of his death so suddenly was heartbreaking. I loved him for all those years and will love him forever.

*

LYNN JORDAAN
Lynn's 58-year-old husband Johan
died from esophageal cancer in 2014

Johan died at home, this is what we both felt was the right thing to do. I was working and worked right up till about four weeks before he died. We had an amazing doctor who called me at work and let me know that Johan didn't have much longer to go. I arranged compassionate leave and came home to be with him.

Johan was not happy about the fact that I was home and kept telling me that I would be bored. I had to tell him, I would rather be bored than have him alone in the house when he died!

He just sort of withdrew into himself in those last days. During the last week of his life the doctor came to see him and told him that he would see him on Friday, but it was okay to go before then if he needed to. I was so angry, how dare he give the man permission to die!

After that visit, Johan kept asking us if it was Friday yet. We teased him, asking him why he needed to know when it was Friday? He had every day off, no need to wait for the weekend before he could do things. He smiled and told me Friday was important.

On the Thursday night, I got up to change his IV bags and noted that it was 11:55 p.m. I went about my business, changed the bags and dillydallied around. At midnight I leaned over him, kissed him and told him that it was Friday. I kind of wish I hadn't done that because a minute later he started the labored breathing. I called my daughter and her husband, and we sat with him for a few minutes and decided to call the doctor. We had been told not to call 911 as they would try and resuscitate him and rush him to hospital. I held the phone to my husband so that the doctor could hear his breathing and then he confirmed that yes, Johan was coming to the end of his journey. I was told that this may take some time, so make some tea and just be with him. I sent the kids back to bed, telling them that I would call them if there was any change. Not sure any of us got any more sleep, but that was the way things were, who can sleep when the fabric of your life is being torn apart.

A little later, I called Johan's sister in Zimbabwe, so that she could say goodbye, and then we waited.

I remember that it was garbage day, so to keep myself busy, I took the garbage out. It had snowed in the night and I struggled a bit. My neighbor came out on his way to work and asked me if I was okay, in the language of the most educated sailor, I told him, no I was most definitely not okay and that Johan was dying. The poor man just held out his arms and hugged me for about five minutes and then took my garbage out for me. I will be forever grateful for that hug. No platitudes not saying anything but that hug said all I needed it to say.

Johan died at 12:30 p.m. that day, it was quiet and peaceful, we were all there with him. My daughter, her husband, the cats, and I. He just sighed and went on his way.

Johan had stated that he did not want a funeral, he wanted no one to cry for him. Yeah right that was about to happen!

So what we did do for him was have a reception, if you will, at home on the Sunday after his death. It was lovely, there was much laughter and many tears but on the whole, it was memories and jokes and would have made him happy had he been there. We did ask that everyone raise a glass of something to drink for him at 8 p.m. on Tuesday in whatever time zone they may be in. It was poignant to realize that he had friends in almost every time zone and for twenty-four hours there was someone in the world wishing him well.

*

GAIL MARCHESA
Gail's husband John died from
colon cancer in 2009 at age 55

John went on hospice care ten days before his death. I think when he made that choice he felt at peace with it. It was tough watching this unfold. I remember him joking long before he was sick saying, "If I get sick, are you gonna change my diaper?" Who knew?

After a few days of hospice, we needed a hospital bed because he tried to get out of bed to use bathroom and fell and he was very heavy to pick up. Then later, he didn't talk and the catheter was slowing up, which I kept staring at. At one point, I thought he had banged up his leg and side because they were bruised. The nurse said it wasn't bruised but the organs shutting down. What a shock that was. I do remember that we all knew he was going to leave that night and I had checked after midnight if he was still breathing. Why? I think I had to know the correct day he went. Hospice is great and I would always recommend them.

*

HEATHER MCLAUGHLIN
Heather's 35-year-old husband Derek
died from colorectal cancer in 2013

The day of Derek's death was a pretty day, I can say that much. It was cold, though. It was January 31, 2013. Derek was confined to his recliner. I had actually just bought a new one that would move up and down with the push of a button. It was very comfy, so Derek really liked it. He had been in the chair the last two days, not getting out. He had a colostomy bag and bladder bag. He was hooked up to fluids when the hospice nurse or one of our nurse friends came to do that.

Derek had pain medication and we tried our best to keep the pain under control, but we could really never get a handle on it. That remains a hard thing for me to swallow. Early that morning, I called the hospice nurse who came and gave Derek pain meds but they just weren't working. The nurse decided to stay for a while. I called our friend Jay who worked for the local emergency management agency. All of the friends I mention work or volunteer for EMS or fire. Jay put a call in to Union EMS since that is the county we lived in, and they came over to help in whatever way we needed.

At some point, Derek woke up and told me to call his boss John, and asked me to turn off his phone. This was huge. I knew it.

Derek's parents and sister came to the house. More EMS friends starting arriving to help—Jay, Beth, Stephanie, the EMS crew, and others. Derek was semiconscious as we loaded him onto the stretcher and into the ambulance for the forty-five minute drive north to the hospice house in Huntersville, North Carolina.

We had been to the hospice house once before to change meds, so they knew us. We arrived and got Derek into a room, and the social worker sat me down to sign papers. We already had a DNR in place.

At some point the weather turned bad. They were trying to get a subcutaneous line into Derek to administer more medication since his PICC line blew, but they couldn't get the meds mixed up from off site and were giving him meds a different way. He had a medication pump and I kept pushing the button for him, which they said was okay. Someone called my mom and she was on her way. Other EMS friends were on their way, too.

I sat by Derek's bed, paced the halls, cried silently, cried loudly, crumpled to the floor and many other things. I remember looking at Derek's legs which were all black and blue; more black than blue. It looked like his legs and feet were rotting off. This scared me but the staff assured me this wasn't hurting Derek. His body was shutting down and pulling blood from his extremities to his core organs, and it was killing his skin cells. It still sounded like it hurt, but I trusted them because hospice was there to try to make people comfortable.

Derek looked like he was sleeping, and they encouraged me to as well. Family slept, but I couldn't. At some point that morning, Derek's dad and sister went back to our house to clean up and let the dogs out. This is when Derek took his last turn. He started exhibiting Cheyne-Stokes respirations when he would breathe and then not breathe for a time. There were a bunch of EMS people at the hospice house now, all in their class A uniforms. I called Dad and Stacie and asked how fast they could return, knowing our time was now very short. They ended up saying goodbye to Derek through the phone held next to his ear.

A bunch of people were in the room. Derek woke and asked for me. I was behind him and came around to where he could see me and held his hand. I looked up and asked if someone could find our wedding song, "I Need You" by Leann Rimes. Our friend Stephanie found it and I put it on Derek's pillow and played it for us. I held his hand, sang parts of the song.

I said to Derek, "I love you. Remember our wedding? Remember getting caught in my train when we danced? . . . Remember our perfect day? . . . I will be okay. I will take care of Zoey and Rio. It's okay, you can close your eyes now and go to heaven. I love you."

The song ended and Derek took his last breath. I knew it before the nurse did. I kissed him and crumpled to the floor, not able to hold it in anymore. It was morning on January 31, 2013.

I eventually went out of Derek's room to tell the EMS crew that Derek had passed, and the nurses were cleaning him up. They said the crews and trucks were already on their way. They gave me hugs.

I held Derek's teddy bear in my hands and wouldn't put it down. The chaplain took me to a sunroom to talk, and pray for me, Derek, and our family. He also asked questions about Derek so he could say some words to honor him as they were wheeling him out. I didn't fully understand what that meant at the time.

A candle had been lit by the nurses station and an American flag had been placed in honor of the passing. I returned to Derek's room and someone had placed rosemary on the door. I went in and they asked for Derek's clothes. I gave them his clothes. I touched him and jumped, not realizing how fast someone turns cold after they die. Derek felt cold and I felt scared. Derek was dead....how? Why? Make him come back! I totally lost it again. Another piece had sunk in. Derek could really be gone....he was cold. I walked out and returned to the sunroom. I didn't know where else to go.

Stuff was happening all around. The rest of the crew arrived and came to see me, and the mortuary people arrived for Derek. Someone came to get the Tahoe keys to wash it before the parade of lights to bring Derek home. I felt lost.

They said it was time. Derek was in a bag-like thing with his head out. The staff and EMS crew lined the hallway. I walked with Derek. I again put my hand on him in hopes he would be warm. He wasn't. I hated this nightmare. For some reason I walked with my head down. I don't know whether I was tired, guilt-ridden, or just not wanting to make eye contact. I was crying and trying to watch where I was going as we walked to the door. The chaplain said a few words about Derek and us as a family. He also said the fireman's prayer. Derek was loaded into the back of the hearse. The lineup went as follows: K-9 officer, engine, Derek, Tahoe, engine, other cars, police car. In Matthews, North Carolina, where Derek was a firefighter and EMT, we would run lights only on all vehicles to the mortuary. I drove Derek's Tahoe.

At the mortuary, a huge American flag waved in the clear blue sky to honor Derek. It was beautiful. More friends, firefighters and medics were there to meet us. Derek was unloaded and wheeled inside. They said I could see him again at the viewing. That took my breath away. They were taking my husband, I didn't know what to think.

Derek's dad guided me back to the car so we could return to the house, shower, and then come back to handle some things. I still don't know how he was so composed. We stayed with the firefighters and medics for a few minutes and then left. I went home, took a shower, and then went to plan Derek's ceremony. By this time it was 4 p.m. Because Derek was an assistant chief, he was awarded a firefighter's funeral. He had a fire engine red casket, the bells, bagpipes, the last ride on the engine, the works. He deserved it.

*

SUE NOVA
Sue's husband Dana died from
lung cancer in 2012 at age 46

About a week before Dana died, I made sure I called everyone to let them know. If they wanted to see him or say anything to him, now was the time. He was awake, drugged, but still communicating.

May 26 was a Saturday. People were kind of in and out. The kids, and their spouses were at the house. Music played, laughter and food. Someone, including a hospice nurse, was always with him.

May 27, later in the afternoon after most people left, he told me he needed to use the bathroom. My son-in-law helped him into the bathroom but my husband kicked him out and asked for me to be in with him. He did his business and I helped him back to bed. He said he was tired and I told him I loved him. He grinned and turned his head to the side. I said to him, "Don't you turn away from me! You better tell me you love me!"

He turned his head to face me, smiled, looked at me and said, "I love you."

Those were the last words he spoke. He fell into the sleep of the actively dying.

May 28 was quiet. The kids were in and out, his best friend was there. I was able to sleep on and off for a few hours.

On May 29, I was woken up about 7 a.m. by the nurse who said that it looked like time was coming close. It was myself, our two kids, and the hospice angel. I was up at his head whispering to him that I loved him and it was okay for him to go. His breathing was almost imperceptible and then it stopped. I gasped and started crying, and kissed him. He then gasped; apparently he wasn't ready to go yet. We were laughing and crying. The kids told me to shut up and stop talking to him so he could go peacefully.

The nurse said we had a little reprieve so if we wanted food or to shower. Now would be the time. In the meantime, our priest showed up because unknowingly, our friend had called him and told him that Dana had died. So he was surprised when he got there to find Dana still hanging on.

A little later, his breathing became very shallow again and it looked like it was time. I was lovingly reminded to shut up. This time, I was joined by the kids, Dana's best friend, and our priest. Our priest read the prayers for the dying and as he finished the final prayer, my beloved husband took his last breath.

Even though I knew it was coming, that final realization hit me in the chest like a ton of bricks. My husband is dead. DEAD. Dead. Nothing prepares you for that moment. I went numb and felt, literally, sick to my stomach. I feel that now, just reliving that moment. The kids told me that almost immediately after Dana died, our dogs, who were outside sitting under his bedroom window, began to howl a very mournful howl.

On May 29, 2012, at 9:44 a.m., my husband, Dana, took his last breath here on earth.

*

SHERYL POCHEL
Sheryl's husband Brian died from
pancreatic cancer in 2011 at age 43

Brian and I never really talked about him actually dying. I know that in the weeks before his death he talked to other people about him dying, but never me. I don't know why. I can only assume it was because I was his rock and he gained his strength from me, and knew if I crumbled, then he would too. So, he didn't talk to me about dying.

The summer he passed away, the brain tumors were starting to take over. He was having a hard time moving around and was losing the use of his right leg. We finally gave in and got him a wheelchair. One morning he made his way to the bathroom and back. He was stubborn and didn't want to use the wheelchair. He sat down on the bed and realized that he had to go to the bathroom again. I told him that I would get the wheelchair, take him in there, give him his privacy and come get him. When I put the wheelchair next to him, he was so angry that he tried to fling himself into it. Instead, he flung himself into the wall and onto the floor.

Two things happened at that moment. First, I could see mini strokes go across his face—his brain was bleeding. I was terrified he was going to die right there on our bedroom floor in nothing but his underwear and t-shirt. The second was that he fractured his neck. Apparently, he had a tumor in his spine we didn't know was there. He was taken to the hospital in an ambulance, where we were very gently told that if the bleeding didn't stop, Brian would die that night.

The bleeding stopped and he lived seven more weeks. He spent the first three in the hospital because of his broken neck. Much to everyone's surprise, he was improving so they decided to move him to a rehab facility. He spent almost two weeks there as he worked on gaining more mobility. He then had another brain bleed and was taken to the hospital again. He spent two or three days there before I made the very difficult decision to move him to the hospice house.

When Brian woke up in the room in hospice, he looked at me and asked who's house we were in. I held his hand and told him that we were at hospice. A single tear ran down his face. After being there for a week, to everyone's surprise he was doing so well that hospice wanted him to go back to the rehab facility. Can you see why it was impossible to think he would die from this? He just always bounced back from everything. The rehab facility wouldn't take him with his pain pump, so that didn't happen. We spent family time together, my family all came out and we grilled out one night. Brian ate not only his food, but mine as well. Apparently, he really wanted steak sandwiches that night! We watched TV together and talked. I spent as much time with him as I could. It was crazy, being with him and figuring out where our kids would be that night. I spent every other night with him while he was there, his mom spent the other nights with him, I was constantly on the run.

The Wednesday before he died I was with him. He was in and out of wakefulness. He was seeing spirits and he was frightened. At one point, his mom asked me if I was leaving soon, she said she was tired and wanted to go to bed. I stayed for another hour, because there was no way I was leaving until I was ready to do so. In that time I leaned in and whispered to Brian "I love you." He said, "I know you do." Then a couple minutes later he said, "I love you, too." It was the last thing he ever said to me.

The next day I had orientation at school for my kids. I was bound and determined to be there for them but all I remember was floating through the halls in a fog. When it was over I went to hospice, and found that Brian was in a coma. No one had bothered to call me and tell me. I stayed with him from that point on, never leaving his side.

Brian died on Saturday, September 3, 2011, at 10:06 p.m. It was a gray and rainy day. The kids came in that Saturday and said their goodbyes. It was so hard. He didn't look like himself any more. He was gaunt and his breathing was raspy. Our youngest daughter was six at the time, and was afraid of him. She sat on the couch next to my dad for a while, then she moved over and sat next to him on the bed. Eventually, she crawled under the covers and curled up next to him and fell asleep. He was scary looking but he was her dad.

The only time I left Brian's side that day was to go eat. My brother and sister had gotten pizzas. I went to the break room because I hadn't eaten all day. On the way back to Brian's room I told the nurse that I wanted to sleep with him that night. My dad was going to stay with me. As my dad and I walked back to his room, he told me about the breathing changes that happen when someone is dying. When we got back into his room, the nurse asked if I'd like to have her give him some morphine and move him over in the bed in a half hour. I took one look at him and asked her if we had a half hour. I knew the answer.

She moved him over, I climbed into bed with him and wrapped my arms around him. A few minutes later he died. I had my eyes closed, when I opened them, his eyes were open and he was looking at my face. He waited for me. He knew I was there. Though our entire family was in the room they all stayed toward the back and in that moment it was just the two of us, just as it should have been. As I finish writing this, I'm listening to Pandora and the song playing is Pachelbel Canon, which we had played at our wedding. He's still here, not how I want him to be, but he's still here . . .

*

KATHIE SCOTT
Kathie's 57-year-old husband Jim
died from prostate cancer in 2009

Oh, those final days! The hospital admission was on a Sunday night and within four hours of going to the emergency room he forgot me. He simply did not know who I was or that we had been married thirty-seven years.

All week the doctors were administering meds to keep Jim comfortable, doing some testing, and preparing to put a PICC line in. On Saturday, we had another member of the neurology team since it was a weekend, and he told me the line would serve no purpose whatsoever and he didn't know if Jim would survive the weekend. His organs were shutting down but they had neglected to discuss that with me. My husband was not coherent so they certainly had not discussed it with him in my absence.

On Saturday, we contacted hospice. On Monday, we went home. Family gathered at our home knowing it was time to say goodbye. My dearest friend parked herself at our home and put herself completely at my disposal. It honestly was the most support I had received during the entire time, and it was both comforting and irritating.

I still did not think death had come through the door. I thought we could hold it at bay for a few days but on Tuesday morning the hospice nurse noticed the signs that death was imminent and made sure I understood what they were seeing. I had sedated him on Monday night, per their instructions, because he was so agitated. The only time he opened his eyes again was near the end, when I was talking to him. He opened his eyes and looked and me and began breathing more slowly. Tuesday night at 9:59 p.m., he took his last breath and I know this because, in my mind, I needed to know the exact time of death because someone would be asking for the official record. I thought I knew how I would handle this moment but I was so wrong! When there was no more breath, this scream came from inside me, a sound I had never heard before. I remember hearing my daughter yelling to her husband to come and help. I had prepared myself for this for more than five years and it was still such a shock that I thought I might die too.

*

STEVE SHARP
Steve's 51-year-old wife Carolyn
died from melanoma in 2014

During the last weeks of her life, Carolyn was taking larger doses of medicine to control her pain. As a result, she drifted in and out of consciousness before becoming comatose the last seven days of her life. She had many visitors during this time period. There were many tears shed as we anticipated her impending death. I remember seeing the shock on the faces of family and friends as we stood by helplessly.

During this time, myself, family, or friends spent the night with Carolyn so she wasn't alone. The night before she died, I sat beside her and planned her funeral. I told her she was a good wife and mother, and it was okay to go. At 11 p.m. I went home when a dear friend arrived to spend the night with Carolyn. She promised she would call me if Carolyn's death was imminent. Unfortunately, Carolyn passed away suddenly at 5 a.m. before I could return. Our friend called me with the news, crying and apologizing that she couldn't call me in time to get there. I told her I understood, and there was nothing she could have done differently. To this day, I still feel guilty that I wasn't there when she died.

*

DIANNE WEST
Dianne's husband Vern died from
multiple myeloma in 2010 at age 69

Vern's kidneys failed around three years after the myeloma diagnosis, so we added dialysis to our list of things cancer brought into our lives. He spent nearly four hours hooked up to that machine three mornings each week. It was very hard on him and he often had difficult reactions. He also received his chemo treatment once a week, so he had to head to the oncology office just a couple of hours after dialysis ended each Friday. That was a hard eighteen months.

On a Monday in mid-September, I began my normal dialysis day routine of waking Vern at 3:30 a.m. to take his meds, letting him go back to sleep while I got dressed, and then waking him at 4:30 to get him dressed and out the door. He hadn't been feeling well over the weekend—lack of appetite, nausea, confusion, fatigue—but since his feet were swollen, I knew he needed the dialysis treatment. I tried to help him get up out of his recliner but couldn't. I tried everything I could think of to help him get out of that chair. Nothing worked and he didn't seem to even be trying. It felt like he was giving up, and I said so through tears. He complained of pain in his left shoulder blade that wouldn't allow him to put any pressure on that arm. I wanted to call for a transport; he wanted to just be left alone that day and said he would try again the next day. We were at an impasse. So, I made a deal with him that if he was unable to get up the next morning, I would make that call.

I called 911 on Tuesday. Luckily, I had placed a sheet on the chair under Vern. Those six wonderfully kind firefighter/EMTs were able to gently lift him and place him on the gurney. Blood draws and IVs were done in the emergency room and they sent him off for scans, x-rays, and an EKG. They wanted to admit him. Hours passed but there were no rooms and finally, eight hours later, we were transported to a different hospital that had an ICU bed waiting for him. He was on good pain meds and fell asleep during his dialysis treatment.

Cardiologist, nephrologist, neurologist, gastroenterologist, and his infectious disease doctor all visited and every single one of them used this same phrase after explaining what their tests had shown: "and he has extremely serious other conditions." I couldn't help but notice the repetition but when I asked for clarification, they said I needed to have a very honest conversation with his oncologist. But his oncologist didn't work out of this hospital, so talking to him would take a while. Instead, I stepped outside the room and asked his nurse pointblank if they were trying to tell us this was the end. She hesitated, saying it really wasn't her place to have this discussion with me. But she was compassionate and said he was a very sick man and we needed to consider quality of life issues. We talked about hospice and she suggested I meet with the palliative care nurse. I shared all of this with Vern, and he said I needed to make that appointment.

How do you know when it's time to stop everything? The thought had never once entered my mind previously, but on this day I couldn't ignore it. I knew Vern was suffering and recognized that he might have been holding on because I refused to see how things really were.

I met with the palliative care nurse the following morning who shared what the doctors were writing on Vern's chart. She explained there was nothing more they could do, that Vern was very, very ill and could not tolerate any further procedures. He would not survive the surgery to repair his clavicle, which had been eaten away by the cancer and was why he could not get out of the recliner. She noted that many caregivers don't hear that message and want to keep fighting the battle in spite of what that means for the patient. I could not do that to Vern. She called hospice and set up an appointment for us later that day.

I felt divinely led to approach Vern's ICU nurse and then the palliative care nurse, and knew this for sure when I walked out of the palliative care office and saw my dear friend Debbie approaching. Our talk was a very special gift of reassurance that this was the right thing and allowed me to get my emotions under control before talking to Vern. As we were chatting outside his room, Vern's best friend Joe arrived. I know that God brought these wonderful people to us at that very moment.

Joe stayed to visit with Vern so I could run home to shower and pick up the things I would need when we moved to hospice. Vern was alert when I returned and we talked about everything. He assured me this is what he wanted. He was so tired of the fight and the pain and said that he was ready to go home. I asked if he wanted to do hospice at home and he said no, he did not want to die in our home. The biggest question I had was whether dialysis would continue; Vern responded that he wanted to stop it.

The hospice nurse arrived and confirmed that he would not be able to continue dialysis in hospice. We both knew this would mean he would only have a few days. I asked Vern again if that was what he wanted and he nodded yes and said, "Why delay the inevitable? I'm ready." We signed the papers and Vern was transferred to Nathan Adelson Hospice Friday evening.

The days in hospice were peaceful. We were grateful he no longer had those nightly intrusions to check blood pressure and temperature. Pain medication was automatic and kept him comfortable. I stayed with him the entire time. He slept a lot but would wake up at times quite alert and ask questions or recognize someone who was visiting and express his thanks. I spoke to him constantly whether he was sleeping or not, as I believed he could still hear me. At one point, I told him I had asked God to send an angel to watch over him and carry him to Heaven. He asked me how many angels he would need because there had been one over in the corner of the room since we arrived. Vern was not an overtly religious man so this statement surprised and comforted me. I told him I thought one would be just enough.

Vern wasn't eating and his bodily functions had pretty much stopped while he was still in the hospital. He had a Foley catheter and a colostomy and I don't think he moved in the bed once we arrived, other than to hold my hand.

Late Tuesday afternoon, he began making a noise that scared me, so I asked the nurse to come in. She explained this was called the death rattle and that it often occurred during a dying person's final hours. She assured me this was not causing him any discomfort. It did not appear to me that he was in pain, so I gently slid into his bed, wrapped my arms around him and began talking to him. I shared memories of our years together, told him it was okay for him to go, that I would miss him every day of my life, that I would survive, that our son and I would get along and be okay, and that I would love him forever and ever. I just talked quietly to him for the next twelve hours until he took his last breath. I stayed laying there next to him for a while and let my tears flow. When I was ready, I walked out to the nurse to let her know he was gone. She came in to officially call a time of death and told me I could have as much time with him as I needed.

The physical change in Vern's face after he died was dramatic. There was a beautiful calm and peaceful aura surrounding him, and it comforted me greatly. He had experienced peripheral neuropathy due to chemo and loved having me massage his feet each night. Before I left the room, I caressed his feet one last time.

The driver from the mortuary arrived and was waiting outside the room. He said I could stay while he prepared Vern for the transfer, but I chose not to. I had said goodbye to my love, had witnessed that peaceful aura, and didn't want anything to replace that image.

After they left, I collected our belongings from the room and headed to my car. I felt numb and so very, very tired. It was early morning and the sun was just beginning to peek over the horizon but the moon was gloriously huge and beautiful. It felt like a message for me and I embraced it on my drive home.

*

CHAPTER SEVENTEEN

Searching For Comfort

Grief changes us. It sculpts us into someone
who understands more deeply. -ANONYMOUS

When the final breath is drawn, we begin a transition into life without our loved one. The future is filled with unknowns, and we look for comfort and familiarity as we move forward alone. Since losing your loved one, what brings you comfort?

*

JANICE DEL VECCHIO
Janice lost her husband Stephen to bile duct cancer in 2006 at age 47, and her second husband John to pancreatic cancer in 2013 at age 55

Being with friends and family helps. I have my husband John's bathrobe and a couple of his shirts. Wearing them gives me a sense of his presence and the feeling he is hugging me. I also have a good chain with a heart and cross attached. The heart was given to me by my first husband, and the cross by my second husband. I would be heartbroken if I lost either one. I also have traveled quite extensively. I loved traveling with them and they both told me to keep traveling, so I do.

*
CYNTHIA HORACEK
Cynthia's husband Don died from
rectal cancer in 2010 at age 57

When my husband died, my younger daughter sent me a card saying, "I know Dad was your purpose. Maybe I can be your purpose now." I didn't want her to take care of me; I'm the mom and I'm supposed to take care of her. What brings me comfort? My daughters and my grandchildren, and making art has helped a lot. It's been very healing for me. I've done art my whole life. When Don died, for three years I couldn't do anything creative. I found an online art journal group and they sent out a prompt every week. I was healing; now I'm back to painting.

*
MARGARET HUTSELL
Margaret's 77-year-old husband Tom
died from pancreatic cancer in 2016

After my husband died, I took his wedding band from his finger where it had rested for fifty-six years, and took it to a jeweler to solder with my wedding band. Together in life, together in death. Each time I look at them on my own hand now, I feel the comfort of our love. I also slept with a pair of his pajamas for a long while, holding them close to my heart each night as I drift off to sleep. I say the Lord's Prayer each night and really think of the words as I say the prayer. I love to talk about him with family and friends.

*

LYNN JORDAAN
Lynn's 58-year-old husband Johan
died from esophageal cancer in 2014

It started off with keeping things Johan wore most often around me so I could still smell him and then pretend he would be home soon. But then his smell started wearing off and all I could smell was me.

I am lucky enough to have grandchildren whom came into my life after Johan passed. The first munchkin is the image of his grandfather, and while there are bittersweet moments, both children bring a lot of happiness, love, and acceptance that life does indeed go on.

I discovered that meditation gets me through the tough spots. Opening up to my daughter about how I am feeling also helps, because I realize then that she is going through much of what I'm going through, albeit on a different level. I get a lot of comfort speaking to the many people who knew and were friends with him. They all realize now that I'm not made of glass and won't break if they mention his name. We still reminisce about stories and happenings that occurred when he was still here. A lot of happy memories and, yes, some sad ones, but that's what keeps him alive in my soul.

My son-in-law and I once had a discussion about what happens when we die. He and I have very differing views, to say the least, but he said that in his heart he believed that a person will always live on so long as there were people still alive to remember them. That was a huge epiphany, and I will always keep that in the back of my mind.

*

HEATHER MCLAUGHLIN
Heather's 35-year-old husband Derek
died from colorectal cancer in 2013

Since losing Derek, my dogs bring me comfort. About seven months after Derek passed away I got a saltwater fish tank. I could control everything inside it: the fish, coral, all parameters, everything. This brought me comfort, because I could control it when my world was so out of control. In the very early days, having the TV on would bring me comfort because it would bring noise to the house. I could watch some shows that Derek and I watched together, others I could not; it depended on the time of day. Friends also helped, who called and told me that we were going to go do something; which forced me to take a shower. This helped me a lot as well. I found a grief support group of young widows which allowed me to openly cry, you know, that ugly cry you don't want anyone to see. They understood it.

*

SHERYL POCHEL
Sheryl's husband Brian died from
pancreatic cancer in 2011 at age 43

Brian's birthday was November 23. On the first birthday after he died, I took my kids to Build-A-Bear and we each picked out a bear to have made. I had vials of Brian's ashes that I put together and we put them in our bears. Each one of us named our bear something that reminded us of him. My bears name is Calvin. I used to call Brian Calvin, there were two reasons. First, he reminded me of Calvin from Calvin and Hobbes, just kind of naughty and sassy sometimes. Second, my background is in apparel design and Brian was my toughest critic, therefore Calvin Klein. I still sleep with my bear, especially when I'm missing him a little more that day. I also still sleep in a couple of his shirts sometimes just to feel close to him.

Brian had a diary. He didn't write in it often, which makes me sad, but what he did write he wrote to the kids. I used that same diary to write to him after he died. It just felt right.

I have also written a blog, though I haven't done it in quite a while. I found it very cathartic to write what was on my mind, and now I can look back on that woman and see how strong she was even though I didn't feel like it at the time. I miss writing. I guess I should start again.

*

KATHIE SCOTT
Kathie's 57-year-old husband Jim
died from prostate cancer in 2009

Comfort? I'm not sure there has been much other than time. I had so often heard or read that the smell from clothes or a pillow would be comforting but I couldn't find that smell. I screamed at cancer more times than I can count that it even robbed him of his scent. I cherished everything he touched or used for a time and slowly I began letting go of objects. It took me a year probably to change anything in his bathroom and more time to empty anything from the closets. Just seeing his belongings brought pain but not to see them would bring more.

My husband died three weeks before Thanksgiving, leaving our holiday rituals with a huge gaping hole. It was now my responsibility to comfort our kids and grandchildren, and hope the empty plate at the holiday table would not be so obvious. Over time, I've returned to hanging the Christmas ornaments we collected during our life, and the memories associated with them are now warm and no longer a sharp pain. Jim wore a scarf wrapped around his neck every winter for forty years, and was well known for this red and blue striped marker. The second year, I was able to put our tree up with our beloved ornaments, but it was missing something. Out comes the red and blue scarf, and has wrapped the top of the tree every year since.

The first birthday after his death was celebrated at the cemetery with Starbucks and we try to have Mexican food around that time because these were such favorites of his. While they were painful at first, they have now become memories that make us smile and encourage happy conversation. I can now talk about him and smile—most of the time. I know it sounds so trite but time really is the great healer. Has it made me well? It has not, but it has provided some measure of comfort.

*

STEVE SHARP
Steve's 51-year-old wife Carolyn
died from melanoma in 2014

I discovered many things that brought me comfort. Our family had requested in Carolyn's obituary that instead of sending flowers to the funeral, people were invited to make a donation to the scholarship fund established in her name to be awarded to two students from the high school where she taught who planned to study chemistry.

Prior to her death, her best friend took Carolyn's thumbprint to use in a jewelry remembrance. On my first birthday after her death, her best friend gave me one on a chain. I added Carolyn's wedding band and a 14k gold replica of her signature and wore it for months. On the first anniversary of her death, Carolyn's family and best friends gathered at the beach, her favorite place, to share memories. We had a brief ceremony at sunrise and even though I had carefully prepared my remarks, I could only get a few words out.

It took a while, but after three years I now find joy in listening to our favorite songs, and remembering the good times associated with the music. Seeing something good come out of a tragedy, helped my outlook and promoted healing. It takes time.

*

DIANNE WEST
Dianne's husband Vern died from
multiple myeloma in 2010 at age 69

In the months after Vern died, I gave myself permission to do whatever I needed to do that felt comforting. Stay up late reading widow blogs. Having a glass of wine before going to bed. Not answering the phone or the doorbell on the weekends. Stay in my jammies on my days off. Sleep in his hospital bed. Okay, that last one even got a reaction from my online bereavement group. But it felt right for me at the time and it certainly wasn't hurting anyone. I wasn't depressed; it was just comforting for me to sleep where he had slept in his final months. I took the hospital bed down at about the two-month mark. Yes, it was after comments were made. But I was ready. If I had wanted to keep sleeping there, I would have regardless of what anyone thought or said. Since then, I've also slept in his recliner whenever the mood strikes and I sleep in his old t-shirts.

Time does soften the pain of loss, but the missing remains and triggers can hit at any time, even many years down the road. When they do, I think it's important to give myself the grace to do whatever brings me comfort. I don't stay in that space for long, just enough to acknowledge it, perhaps write about it, and then pull myself back up to face the day.

The mortuary gave me a small sealed bag of ashes separate from the urn which I carry with me whenever I travel. It makes me feel good to bring him along on my travels. On those really hard days, that little bag brings me great comfort by just holding it close to my heart.

I purchased a photo locket necklace that has Vern's photo on the front and our wedding kiss photo on the back that I wear all the time. Sometimes I wear it under my clothes, most of the time it's in full view. It's just another little thing that keeps him close to me. It's teardrop-shaped and has a very smooth surface and I'll often just hold it in my hand during special moments like a blessing stone.

I've worn Vern's wedding band on my left hand since it flew off his finger in the hospital. He liked seeing it there since he couldn't wear it any longer. I wore it with my rings for several years but now I just wear his band and a widow's ring. I've had people ask why I still wear his ring on my left hand. I usually reply that since I don't want to date it just makes it easier, but really? Why on earth should anyone care whether I wear his ring or which hand it is on? I also have a simple silver ring with Vern's name stamped on it that I wear on my right hand. It's important to me to continue to say his name and this ring and the pendant often provide that opportunity. I feel very strongly that there are no rules about how we should grieve, and no one has the right to tell us we are doing it wrong.

I started doing random acts of kindness (RAKs) on our wedding anniversary three years ago and what a wondrous comfort that brings me each year on a day that previously had been so hard to get through. That first year was for our forty-fifth wedding anniversary, so I came up with forty-five things to give out. Donuts for the emergency room and nursing staff at the hospital he spent the most time in; gift cards for the nurses to hand out to patients who needed them; flowers presented to patients on the surgical and oncology floors; balloons with a love note attached to cars in the emergency lot. It was a magical morning for our son, Jeremy, and I to experience the surprise and gratitude of those we met.

The next year, the fifth anniversary of Vern's death, hit me rather hard, so I didn't spend the day delivering RAKs. Instead, I wrote little love notes and later slid them inside books at the library, between cans in the grocery store, or handed to a cashier at the drive-through.

Last year, I put together packages of socks, a love note, a little heart token, and five dollars, and gave them out to the homeless people I encountered. I've actually continued to keep a basket of these in my car to give out all year long. Each of these RAKs includes a little card with Vern's name on it and it brings me great comfort to be doing something kind and unexpected for others in his memory.

*

CHAPTER EIGHTEEN

Seeking Hope

Be like the birds, sing after every storm.
-BETH MENDE CONNY

Losing someone we love has a way of redefining hope for each of us. Since losing a loved one to cancer, what is your definition of hope?

*

JANICE DEL VECCHIO
Janice lost her husband Stephen to bile duct cancer in 2006 at age 47, and her second husband John to pancreatic cancer in 2013 at age 55

To me, hope means the promise of a new day. When you have a particularly bad day, there's always tomorrow. I try to live a meaningful life and experience as much as I can.

*

CYNTHIA HORACEK
Cynthia's husband Don died from
rectal cancer in 2010 at age 57

My definition of hope is to be able to look toward the future and believe there is something good there. It's hard to have hope when you're alone and the love of your life is gone. But without hope, what do we have? I have to hope for the future; for the future of my grandchildren and that they will still have a viable earth to live on. So I hope—I hope for our democracy, for the planet, and for all the children here.

*

MARGARET HUTSELL
Margaret's 77-year-old husband Tom
died from pancreatic cancer in 2016

My hope is to find a new focus in life. I am still drifting, and need and want to find new friends who are widows or widowers who know what I'm feeling. I need someone to go out to coffee with, lunch dates or a movie—anything to bring a smile to my heart. I hope I can make the big move into a smaller home and not feel like I am abandoning Tom. He died at home, in our bed and moving might make me start to move on from him. I am frightened by that.

*

LYNN JORDAAN
Lynn's 58-year-old husband Johan
died from esophageal cancer in 2014

My definition of hope it is that while the sun rises in the morning, there is a new day to do some good, a new beginning, if you will. There will be rough days, but I've to live that rough day only for the moment. I'll ride the wave until it meets the shore and peters out. The next wave won't be as high or long as the last. The next will bring a glimmer of happy with it. Tomorrow will be a happy day.

*

HEATHER MCLAUGHLIN
Heather's 35-year-old husband Derek
died from colorectal cancer in 2013

As I continue to move through my journey my vision of hope changes. As soon as Derek passed away, my definition of hope was holding onto all the ties that I could; regardless of whether they were social, physical, material, immaterial, it didn't matter. As life happened, some of those ties broke down and that was very difficult, but I learned that not everyone wants to remember the same way and at the same time. This was a hard lesson for me to learn since Derek was so active in fire/EMS.

At about six months after Derek passed away, I moved myself and our dog, Rio, to Arizona, to try to get away from the sorrowful stares and the "I am so sorry," that surrounded my life. Since Derek was so well known, I couldn't go anywhere without someone knowing me, and feeling like that widowed mark was always hanging over me. I felt like I couldn't grieve the way I needed to where I was currently living. I was offered a job in Flagstaff, Arizona, and moved two thousand miles away from anyone I ever knew. Brave and scary. My mom and friends packed up my house, I really couldn't. Whenever I came across something of Derek's, it would send me spiraling. Sometimes I could deal with it, most of the time, I couldn't.

My mom and I made the trip and spent a lot of time talking about how to stay brave and learn how to be an adult again. At that point my vision of hope was the fact that I had to and knew I could do it on my own. About five months after I got to Flagstaff, I found and bought a house on my own, which was huge! I restocked my fish tanks and was doing well at my HS teaching job. Hope had moved from surviving the minute to surviving the day, to now looking at wanting to adopt children…I wanted a family! My hope had shifted back to the future. In November 2015, I met the practicum teacher in Physics next door, Matthew. We were cordial to each other and in December 2015 he asked for my number and we got lunch. Things developed from there and we started dating. We dated, had a quick engagement, and were married on March 17, 2017. My hope now has my new husband and our future family in it. It will always have Derek in it, but I know that this is what Derek would have wanted for me.

*

SHERYL POCHEL
Sheryl's husband Brian died from
pancreatic cancer in 2011 at age 43

I had a mantra while Brian was sick, and that was hope, believe, dream. I hoped for his survival and better days, I believed it could happen, and I dreamed of our future. That is what hope meant to me then. Now, this is what it looks like to me: Hold. On. Pain. Ends.

This is one of my definitions. While the pain doesn't end, it does certainly get better with time.

I am in a much different place than I was six years ago. I have hope again. The severest of the pain has diminished and I'm left with the possibilities of my future. That is a good place to be.

*

KATHIE SCOTT
Kathie's 57-year-old husband Jim
died from prostate cancer in 2009

I knew I could never give up hope that there would be some miracle and cancer would not take my husband from me and my children's father from them. In holding onto this particular thread, I think I did all of us a disservice. We knew the cancer could not be removed and would not be cured and would eventually take his life. If I could go back in time and take this journey over I would keep my hope in perspective. My hope would be in small pieces and not one big grand picture. I would hope for a good day, a loving moment shared with complete honesty, a release of emotions on an as needed basis. Hope would not be to fight this monster knowing it had insurmountable ammunition. Hope would be to have the best day we could possibly have without thought for what tomorrow might bring.

*

STEVE SHARP
Steve's 51-year-old wife Carolyn
died from melanoma in 2014

It is all too easy after the loss of a loved one to look at the world harshly. The hope I had for my loved one to beat cancer wasn't realized. It could have easily left me bitter and angry.

Today my hope is that people will remember Carolyn, not as a cancer victim, but as someone special who dedicated her life to her family and teaching young people to achieve their goals and believe in themselves. I sincerely hope that people will believe that having known my wife, their world is a better place.

*

DIANNE WEST
Dianne's husband Vern died from
multiple myeloma in 2010 at age 69

I've always been a pretty positive and hope-filled person, looking on the bright side of things and expecting good things to happen. And when they didn't, well, I tried to find the lesson to be learned during those hard times. Sometimes it takes a while to discover it, but you won't find it unless you seek it. I'll admit that there were times during those cancer years that I really struggled to understand the why of everything that happened but I never truly lost hope. Hope for me was a belief that something good was going to happen...hope that he would survive that particular crisis, hope that I would be able to bring him home, hope that I would endure the stress. And when we headed to hospice? It was hope that he would be pain-free, hope that his passing would be peaceful, hope that I would find the best way to comfort him, hope that I would survive living without him.

And now that I am alone, hope is what keeps me going. Hope that I'm on the right path, hope that I'm making a difference, hope that Vern is proud of me and the choices I'm making.

Hope matters...it truly does. And believing that good things can—and will—happen in the midst of our sorrow makes such a difference in our lives.

CHAPTER NINETEEN

Making Peace with the Journey

Sometimes you have to go through things,
and not around them. -ANONYMOUS

Every journey is as unique as one's fingerprint, for we experience different beliefs, desires, and needs. Though we may not see anyone else on the path, we're never truly alone, for more people walk behind, beside, and in front of us. What would you like the world to know about your journey?

*

JANICE DEL VECCHIO
Janice lost her husband Stephen to bile duct cancer in 2006 at age 47, and her second husband John to pancreatic cancer in 2013 at age 55

Taking care and losing two husbands seem surreal to me now. My advice regarding my experiences is to try to not make any big decisions while you are in the beginning stages of grief. It's easy to have a knee jerk reaction when you are stressed to the max. Some decisions have to be made initially but not your entire life. If you are lucky, you spend a big part of your life with your husband and to think you have to make all kinds of decisions is not true. You need time to digest the fact that you are uncoupled. I had a widowed friend tell me it was okay not to do things you don't want to do. Great advice. Best example is learning to say no. Also, I advise getting grief counseling at some point in your grief journey. It's helpful in that you can talk to someone who doesn't know you or your story. I was dropped out of social situations when I became widowed both times. It was hard but I learned to make new friends with people who understood my situation and kinder and gentler human beings. Sometimes, you have to walk away from relationships that become toxic. People will constantly slide in and out of your life. It was hard to figure that out but you will learn to realize when it is time to let go. You need to tend to your needs now and children if you have them.

*

CYNTHIA HORACEK
Cynthia's husband Don died from
rectal cancer in 2010 at age 57

I would like others to know that you cannot give up hope until it is unequivocally gone. When you get that final prognosis in terms of "There's nothing else we can do," and how much time your loved one has left, you cannot give up. My husband never gave up until that final prognosis, and then he told our daughter that in a way it was a relief, that he could stop fighting. I took off from work to be with him when he was diagnosed and I'm so glad I did. We made the most of that last year, even when we thought he'd beat it; we didn't put anything off that he was well enough to do. At first there's a numbness and you're busy taking care of paperwork and getting everything in order. When the numbness wears off, usually that's when people are gone and you are truly alone. But you have to just get through it; you have to allow yourself to grieve and cry and rant and rave when you need to. You have to not hold back or hold it in. And you need to not apologize to anyone for how you feel. Grief is a process, you can't get over it or under it; you go through it and each one of us has our own process. Grief has no timeline and there are no nice, neat stages. It just happens. My husband has been gone seven years as I write this. I miss his as much today as I did when I first lost him. I will always miss him.

*

MARGARET HUTSELL
Margaret's 77-year-old husband Tom
died from pancreatic cancer in 2016

Our fourteen-month journey with cancer was an icing on the cake period of time. Even though we knew from day one that Tom's chances of surviving were tiny, we continued to get up each morning, thanking God we had each other and could spend another twenty-four hours together. We talked about everything, we did exactly what we wanted to do, and when we wanted to do it. We saw and visited only with those we wanted to be with. Our bucket list contained one wish, and that was to spend each day together until Tom's last breath.

Like many other couples who are together for as long as we were, we had thought we had at least ten to fifteen more good years together. We moved through life as though nothing could interfere with our plans. God was probably smiling and wondering why we were so naïve. Live life each and every day you have. Nothing is promised, and there is never enough time when you truly love someone.

We felt supported by our medical community, our family, most of our friends and were touched by their sensitivity to our situation. This wasn't our plan, but clearly God had other plans in place for us. I kept telling Tom I would be all right and he needn't worry about me. Little did I know, even with fourteen months to prepare, how truly devastating his passing would be. It is what it is, and I know things will be okay down the line. It just hurts like hell.

*

LYNN JORDAAN
Lynn's 58-year-old husband Johan
died from esophageal cancer in 2014

I think the best advice to anyone starting this journey is to embrace the feelings, know that the tsunami will only last so long before the storm water recedes. Yes, there will be another wave, and maybe the new one will be as bad as the last, but the time between the waves will stretch out longer and longer.

There will come a time when you look out the window and see that the sky is blue, hear the birds singing, and you actually feel good. I think that this will take longer for some than others, but each journey is so different, much like anything in life.

Reach out to other people who have experienced loss, you will find a community out there.

Don't expect friends and family to always understand what you are going through. Life goes on for them too, and their responsibilities may get in the way of them being there for you.

Also, people say dumb things. Try not to be offended, they know not what they are doing, they have been lucky so far in their lives and have no clue what it is like to lose a part of themselves.

Most of all know that you are loved. God Bless.

*

HEATHER MCLAUGHLIN
Heather's 35-year-old husband Derek
died from colorectal cancer in 2013

The word cancer, it's an ugly word, it's a scary word. Don't let someone, not even a doctor, tell you or your significant other that it is wrong to take antidepressants or anxiety meds. Get them prescribed if you need them. Cancer is a messy process, from beginning to end and afterwards.

Get the answers you need. If it doesn't make sense, ask again. I wish we would have done that at the beginning of the 5-FU treatment and after he came out of the Cleveland Clinic surgery, after we learned it was terminal and countless other times. There doesn't seem to be enough time to let it all sink in. I can't stress enough to ask questions.

Don't always put on a good face for your significant other. Most of the time, they are struggling just as much as you are. Derek finally told me this and we had some good conversations where we just grieved together of things cancer took from us before he passed away. Those moments are powerful.

We pushed away some friends not knowing what to tell them when they wanted to help. I wish we would have just accepted the help of dog walking, food, respite for me and anything else they were offering. I got very run down trying to do it all, even after Derek's death. Let people help you.

Eat. I lost so much weight because I was busy, scared, you name it. I can remember my mom making a small grilled cheese sandwich and just setting it beside me after Derek passed away. I had not eaten in a day or so, and she said, "Just in case you might be hungry." It ended up smelling good, so I took a few bites and ate the sandwich. Stay hydrated too with water, Gatorade, whatever you have.

Be gentle to yourself. This one I know you have heard. It's true though. Some ways that I was gentle to myself: went for walks outside, rocked on the hammock, swung on my swings (on my swing set), curled in Derek's clothes or blanket, or went to Derek's firehouse or a live burn training exercise. I tried to read, but it took me three years to finally finish reading a book cover to cover. I colored a lot too, that always helped my nerves and made me concentrate on other things. Whatever it is, make sure it makes you smile (even a little), because that is important. Don't forget to talk about your significant other too, that is also very important. I try and tell a story everyday about Derek.

*

SHERYL POCHEL
Sheryl's husband Brian died from
pancreatic cancer in 2011 at age 43

One of the first things I did after Brian died was to join a young widows support group in my area. I had this theory, the sooner I got myself into something grief related the sooner that pain would go away. Ha! Boy was I wrong! It did help though because I didn't feel alone, and I still go to those meetings monthly.

I also started going online to a site called Widowed Village. There was a round-the-clock chat room there and it was comforting to know that there was always someone on the other end that understood what I was going through. I met one of my closest friends on there. It turned out that we live less than a half hour away from each other and we are extremely close. Widowed Village led me to Camp Widow, which is the single best thing I could have ever done for myself. The healing that happens in that weekend is nothing short of amazing. I've actually gone several times, and look forward to going again. Being with other widowed people who "get it" is the best. I don't feel so alone.

Living through, and past, my husband's cancer was the hardest thing I have ever had to do, and I hope I never have to do it again. It shaped me into who I am today, and that is a much different person than I was when he was diagnosed. I'm strong, not because I want to be, but because strong was the only choice I had. Brian would be proud of me. He would love how I am raising our kids, I believe he would like the man who is my partner and how he treats me and our kids, he would be impressed with my weight loss and how I look now and he would be proud of the fact that I am starting my own business. All of that gives me comfort. I still live my life with his shadow. I take what I learned from him and pay it forward. I still love him as much as I did the day he died, and not only is that okay, it feels good. I'm so very lucky to have had him in my life for twenty-five years. Our relationship shaped me from a teenager into an adult, and his death reshaped me into who I am today. Even in death he is a factor in my life, and I wouldn't have it any other way. Long live love.

*

KATHIE SCOTT
Kathie's 57-year-old husband Jim
died from prostate cancer in 2009

I have been through several cancer journeys with family members. My husband and my sister were my lifelines and the two people in the world who were always holding me up and supporting me. As I have said, my husband and I didn't talk much about what would happen and how we would handle the rough times and the end. I didn't want to talk about it, because that meant I had no hope and had accepted that cancer would win. This has caused me much pain and guilt since his death. I wish we would have openly discussed the fact that he was going to die. He tried many times to open the door and I slammed it shut every time. This must have caused him a lot of frustration and pain and that is hard for me to reconcile. When my sister knew she had very little time left, she talked to me about her choice to not have treatments. She was ready to die. I learned from my past and allowed her to talk about it, and I accepted it. I have not suffered nearly as much with her death because I allowed her to give me this gift of acceptance. If I could give a family one piece of advice, it would be to have open and honest discussions and share your feelings. It might seem painful in the moment but in the long term, it will be a tremendous source of comfort for everyone.

*

STEVE SHARP
Steve's 51-year-old wife Carolyn
died from melanoma in 2014

The support that I got from family and friends during Carolyn's struggle with cancer was a godsend. I learned that there is nothing wrong with accepting help from people. Receiving help doesn't mean that you are a weak person. Instead, it is gracefully allowing others to walk with you and help carry your burden. It became clear to me that it was also a blessing to those giving support as they too loved Carolyn.

I became active in a support group for those who lost their spouse which was extremely helpful. This group was facilitated by leaders who had experienced a similar loss. I also found Camp Widow online and attended two events. These were very positive experiences for me and I highly recommend them.

With time I came to understand that I was blessed to have been married to a wonderful woman who loved me until the day she died. The greater tragedy would have been not to have known Carolyn and experienced her love.

Finally, because of the vital support I received, I recently decided to complete training as a local grief group facilitator. This gives me the opportunity to give back to others what I have found to be so helpful.

Time heals but the only way that happens is if you really work at it. I am a work in progress.

*

DIANNE WEST
Dianne's husband Vern died from
multiple myeloma in 2010 at age 69

Cancer sucks. Sorry to be blunt, but it's true. The cancer journey is a hard one, different for each patient and caregiver, but so very hard. It's easy to fall into the "Why me? Why us?" rabbit hole, but that really does not help. Learning that you are not alone will make a difference. Please believe that. Find your tribe. Find people either locally or online who share your story. Look for a group of patients or caregivers who are fighting the same cancer. If you've lost your love, seek out other widowed people. Try some local groups. If they don't feel right for you, don't feel obligated to keep attending, just move on to the next one. And if you can't find one, consider starting one of your own. Connecting with others who know what you're going through, who are either farther down the road or coming up from behind, will change your life. Trust me.

Finding things to be grateful for, even on really hard days, will make a difference. It wasn't always easy to come up with things each day. At the beginning it might have just been, "I got dressed today," or

"I put clean sheets on the bed." Soon I was able to hear the birds chirping outside my window or appreciate the beauty of the full moon. Make an effort to look for something positive, something you can be thankful for every single day, and you will start to see it all around you. It will make a real difference.

On May 4, 2006, I began the hardest journey of my life. I had no idea where it would lead, what it would hold, or when it would end. The only thing I knew for sure was that I would stand by my husband through it all, no matter what came our way. And I did. And that's all that you can do, too. Be kind to yourself. Give yourself a grace card whenever you need to. You may regret some things along the way; I sure did. But just keep love as your guiding theme and all will be well. Love yourself. Love your person. Even love your medical team.

The medical system can leave much to be desired these days. Doctors. Nurses. Technicians. Medical office staff. They are human and mistakes will unfortunately happen. Hopefully, those errors will be rather inconsequential. Some, however, could be life-threatening. Being your loved one's advocate is critical, but is very hard work. Stay the course while you're in the midst of it. Choose to spend your time and energy on what is most important. Use your tribe to help you ask the right questions and know what you should expect.

You will survive this, I promise. Some patients will survive it, too. But if your loved one does not, please know that you will survive that devastating loss, too. There are many of us waiting to hold your hand as you take those steps back into your life.

I knew I had to find something to give my life purpose after Vern died. It would have been easy for me to just go to work and then come home and grieve in silence. But that would not have been healthy and it would not have honored the life I shared with Vern. So I started seeking things I could do and places I could go that would open new doors for me.

I found Widowed Village (widowedvillage.org) that connected me to other widowed people. That led me to attend Camp Widow where I met many of my online widowed friends along with many others. Interacting with those who were further along in their grief gave me hope that I would get there, too (www.campwidow.org).

I started volunteering for Soaring Spirits International, a non-profit organization that hosts the Widowed Village site and Camp Widow weekends, and I now serve as their volunteer coordinator and manage the Widowed Village web site. I also oversee the forty-plus regional social groups across North America that meet in their local areas to support widowed people, and have started a group in my own community. Giving back has made an important difference in my life (www.soaringspirits.org).

I also looked for creative things to help me heal. I took online art classes, started writing a blog, went to some art retreats. I enjoyed some; others not so much. But the important thing was that I was putting myself out there. Facing life head on to find my purpose. I found Brave Girls Club (bravegirlsclub.com) and it offered online soul work and art classes that helped me heal. I recently trained with them to become a certified instructor for their Soul Restoration course and have started holding women's retreats where I teach that curriculum.

I never saw any of this in my future before Vern died. Our dream was to travel the world in our retirement. But that option was taken away, so I needed to find something that would help me honor him, to honor the years we spent together. Locking myself inside our home and withdrawing from life was just not an option. I hope that you will agree that is not an option for you either and that you will actively seek out what your heart needs to begin to heal.

*

The sky takes on shades of orange during sunrise
and sunset, the color that gives you hope
that the sun will set only to rise again.

RAM CHARAN
*

Finding the Sunrise

One night after my daughter died in a car accident, I had a vivid nightmare. I was running frantically toward a sunset, trying to catch it before it descended below the horizon. From behind me was the approaching pitch-black abyss of nightfall. Terrified of the darkness, I ran as fast as my legs could carry me away from the abyss and toward the setting sun, but it wasn't fast enough. In spite of my efforts, the sun's warm light sank out of my reach.

Dreams have a way of revealing a message, and this one was clear: if I wanted to see the sun ever again, I had to stop running toward a sunset I couldn't catch. For just as there would be no rainbow without the rain, the sun only rises on the other side of night. I had no choice but to turn around and walk head-on into the gaping nightfall of grief. Then—and only then—would I find my way through to the other side.

I remember reading that if I didn't allow myself to experience the full scope of my grief, it would come back to bite me. I couldn't fathom how it could get any worse but knew I didn't want to test that theory. I gave in and allowed the grief to swallow me whole. I wailed on my daughter's bedroom floor. I penned my deep emotions, regardless who might read it. I created a national radio show to discuss our journeys with anyone who wanted to call in. And I allowed myself to sink to the bottom of the fiery pits of hell. But sitting in the belly of hell for the rest of my life wasn't an option. I was too young. I had to find a way out of the hole or die trying.

Today, I'm often asked how I manage my grief so well. Some assume that because I found peace and joy, I'm avoiding my grief. Others believe that because I work in the bereavement field, I'm wallowing in self-pity. Well, which is it? Neither. I miss my child with every breath I take. Just like you, I will always have my moments and triggers: the painful holidays, birthdays, death anniversaries, a song or smell that evokes an unexpected memory. But I've also found purpose, beauty, and joy again. It takes hard work and determination to over-come profound grief, and it also takes the ability to let go and succumb to the journey. Do not be afraid of the tears, sorrow, and heartbreak; after all, they are a natural reaction—and imperative to healing.

There is a vast assortment of tools to help you along the journey, each created by someone who walked in your shoes and understands the heartache. Collect a toolbox of bereavement tools, and avail yourself to whatever tools feel best. Many wonderful resources are available, but what brings comfort to one might irritate the next. Bereavement tools are not one-size-fits-all, so if one tool doesn't work, find another.

Grief is not something we get over. It's a journey through re-building of self. But it is survivable, those who have walked before us are proof. And if they've survived, why not me? Why not you?

On the following pages are the baby steps I took to put hell in my rearview mirror and find the sunrise on the other side. At first each step took great effort and lots of patience, but like any dedicated routine it got easier over time. And the reward of finding balance in my life was worth every step.

1. VALIDATE YOUR EMOTIONS

The first step is to validate your loss. When we talk about our deep heartbreak, we aren't ruminating in our sorrow or feeling sorry for ourselves. Discussing it allows us to process it. If we aren't allowed to process it, then it becomes silent grief. Silent grief is deadly grief.

Find a friend who will patiently listen to you for fifteen minutes every day. Set the timer, and ask him or her not to say anything during those fifteen minutes. Explain that it's important for you to just ramble without interruption, guidance, or judgment. You need not have the same listener each time, but practice this step <u>every</u> day.

2. COMPASSIONATE THOUGHTS

Find yourself a quiet spot. It can be your favorite chair, in your car, in your office, or even in your garden. Then clear your head and for five minutes think nothing but compassionate thoughts about yourself. Not your spouse, not your children, not your coworkers, but yourself. Having trouble? Fill in the blanks below, and then give yourself permission to really validate those positive qualities. Do this every day.

I have a ____

Example: good heart, gentle soul, witty personality

I make a ____

Example: good lasagna, potato salad, scrapbook, quilt

I'm a good____

Example: friend, gardener, knitter, painter, poem writer

People would say I'm ____

Example: funny, kind, smart, gentle, generous, humble, creative

3. TENDER LOVING CARE

While grieving, it is important to consider yourself as being in the intensive care unit of Grief United Hospital, and treat yourself accordingly. How would nurses treat you if you were their patient in the ICU? They would be compassionate, gentle, and allow for plenty of rest. That is exactly how you should treat yourself. Also, consider soothing your physical self with tender loving care as an attentive way to honor your emotional pain. This doesn't mean you have to book an expensive massage. If wearing fuzzy blue socks offers a smidgen of comfort, then wear them unabashedly. If whipped cream on your cocoa offers a morsel of pleasure, then indulge unapologetically.

Treating our five senses to anything that offers a perception of delight might not erase the emotional heartache, but it will offer a reminder that not all pleasure is lost. List five ways you can offer yourself tender loving care, and then incorporate <u>at least three</u> into your day, every day. With practice, the awareness of delight eventually becomes effortless, and is an important step toward regaining joy.

TLC suggestions:

- Shower or bathe with a lovely scented soap
- Soak in a warm tub with Epsom salts or a splash of bath oil
- Wear a pair of extra soft socks
- Light a fragrant candle and listen to relaxing music
- Apply a rich lotion to your skin before bed
- Indulge in a few bites of your favorite treat
- Enjoy a mug of your favorite soothing herbal tea
- Add whipped cream to a steaming mug of cocoa

4. SEE THE BEAUTY

Listening to the birds outside my bedroom window every morning was something I had loved since childhood. But when Aly died, I found myself deaf and blind to the beauty around me. My world had become colorless and silent. One morning as I struggled to get out of bed, I halfheartedly noticed the birds chirping outside my bedroom window. My heart sank as I realized that they had been chirping all along, but I was now deaf to their morning melody. Panic set in as I concluded that I would never enjoy life's beauty ever again. Briefly entertaining thoughts of suicide to escape the profound pain, I quickly ruled it out. My family had been through so much already; I couldn't dump further pain on them. But in order to survive the heartbreak, I had to find a way to allow beauty back into my life. So on that particular morning as I lay in bed, I forced myself to listen and really <u>hear</u> the birds. Every morning from that point forward, I repeated that same exercise. With persistent practice, it became easier and then eventually effortless to appreciate the birds chirping and singsongs. Glorious beauty and sounds have once again returned to my world.

Profound grief can appear to rob our world of all beauty. Yet despite our suffering, beauty continues to surround us. The birds continue to sing, flowers continue to bloom, the surf continues to ebb and flow. Reconnecting to our surroundings helps us to reintegrate back into our environment.

Begin by acknowledging one small pleasantry each day. Perhaps your ears register the sound of singing birds or you notice the sun's radiance on a red rosebush. Give yourself permission to notice one pleasantry, and allow it to <u>really</u> register.

Here are some suggestions:

- Listen to the birds sing (hearing)
- Visit a nearby park and listen to the children (hearing)
- Notice the pretty colors of blooming flowers (sight)
- Light a fragrant candle (scent)
- Attend a local recital, concert, play, or comedy act (hearing)
- Wear luxury socks (touch)
- Wrap yourself in a soft scarf or sweater (touch)
- Enjoy a Hershey's chocolate kiss (taste)

5. PROTECT YOUR HEALTH

After our daughter's death, I soon found myself fighting an assortment of viruses which compounded my frazzled emotions. Studies show that profound grief throws our body into "flight or fight" syndrome for months and months, which is very hard on our physical bodies. It becomes critical to guard our physical health. Incorporating a few changes into our daily routine feels hard at first, but soon gets easy. Plus, a stronger physical health helps to strengthen our coping skills.

Below are a few suggestions to consider adding to your daily routine to help your physical self withstand the emotional upheaval.

- Practice good sleep hygiene
- Drink plenty of water
- Take a short walk outside every day
- Resist simple carbohydrates
- Keep a light calendar, guard your time carefully, and don't allow others to dictate and overflow your schedule

6. FIND AN OUTLET

In the first year, little things like getting out of bed or taking a shower can be exhausting. As painful as it is, it's very important to find an outlet that gets you out of bed each day. Finding something to distract you from the pain, occupy your mind, and soothe your senses can be tricky, but possible. Performing a repetitive action can calm your mood, and even result in a new craft or gifts to give.

Beginning a new outlet may feel exhausting at first, but remember that the first step is always the hardest. And you don't have to do it forever, just focus on it for the time being. Possible activities include:

- Learn to mold chocolate or make soap
- Learn how to bead, knit, crochet, or quilt
- Volunteer at a local shelter
- Learn a new sport such as golf or kayaking
- Create a memorial garden in a forgotten part of the yard
- Join Pinterest
- Doodle, draw or color
- Learn to scrapbook or join a book club

Grief is hell on earth. It truly is. But when walking through hell, your only option is to keep going. Eventually the hell ends, the dark night fades to dawn, and the sun begins its ascent once again.

Just keep going and you, too, will find the sunrise.

Lynda Cheldelin Fell

I already know sorrow.
Today I choose joy.

LYNDA CHELDELIN FELL

255

Meet the writers

One smile can change a day.
One hug can change a life.
One hope can change a destiny.

LYNDA CHELDELIN FELL
*

256

*

JANICE DEL VECCHIO
Janice lost her husband Stephen to bile duct cancer in 2006 at age 47,
and her second husband John to pancreatic cancer in 2013 at age 55
jdvecc@gmail.com

Janice Benedict Del Vecchio is originally from Massachusetts and currently resides in New Hampshire. She shares her home with her cats, Chickpea and Tigger. Janice is an executive assistant to seven investment professionals at Fidelity Investments in Boston. Interests include traveling, swimming, kayaking, snowshoeing, hiking and wine tasting.

*

CYNTHIA HORACEK
Cynthia's husband Don died from
rectal cancer in 2010 at age 57

Cynthia and Don Horacek were married for thirty-one years when Don died from rectal cancer in 2010. Since Don's death, they've had three grandsons added to the one born before Don died, and Cynthia is the proud parent of their two daughters. Cynthia is a retired marriage and family therapist who spends her time volunteering at the local hospital and painting, her first passion (aside from Don).

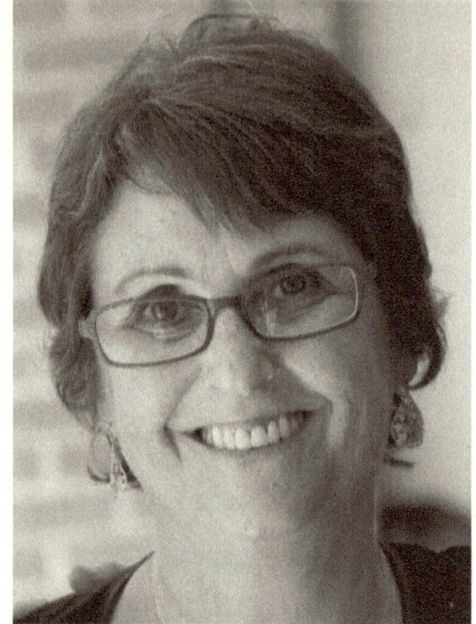

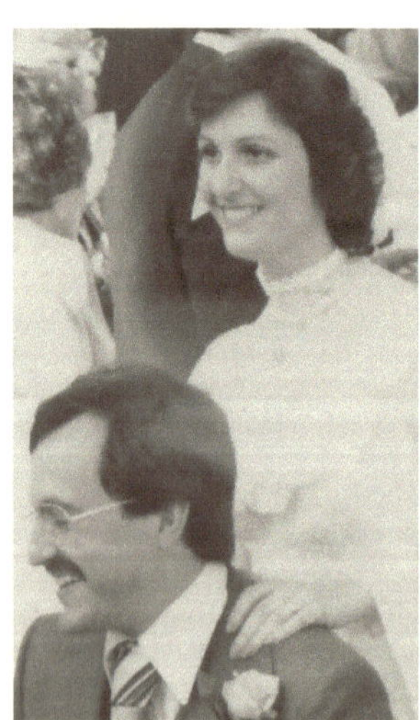

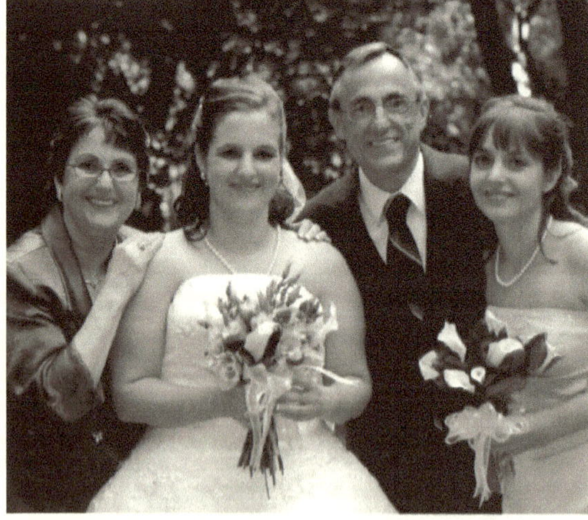

*

MARGARET HUTSELL
Margaret's 77-year-old husband Tom
died from pancreatic cancer in 2016

Marge was born in New Jersey but has lived in the Midwest most of her life. Marge and Tom were married in 1960, and began their family soon after. Marge's passion is her family. Three children, seven grandchildren, and one great-grandchild gave her focus and brought joy and she continues to spend as much time as possible with all of them. Interests include music (from pop to country to classical), reading, writing, playing board games with anyone willing to sit a spell and play, and spending family vacations at the beach in Florida during winter.

The role of caregiver to Tom during his last fourteen months was an honor and privilege and the fifty-seven years they were together was magical.

*

LYNN JORDAAN
Lynn's 58-year-old husband Johan
died from esophageal cancer in 2014

Lynn Jordaan was born in Port Elizabeth, South Africa, and raised in Salisbury, Rhodesia (now Zimbabwe). She spent half her married life in Johannesburg, South Africa, and the rest in Toronto, Canada. She is a mom of one and Grammy of two beautiful little boys.

*

GAIL MARCHESA
Gail's husband John died from
colon cancer in 2009 at age 55

Gail Marchesa is originally from New Jersey, and moved to South Carolina in 2011. She retired from the military in 2009. She lives with five cats and is active with friends.

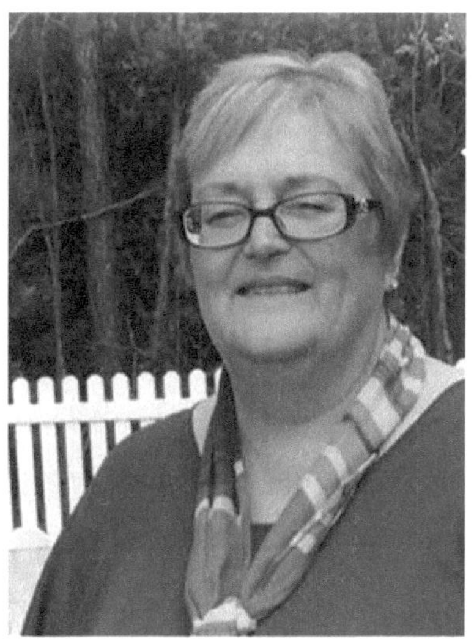

*

HEATHER MCLAUGHLIN
Heather's 35-year-old husband Derek
died from colorectal cancer in 2013

Heather McLaughlin was born in New Jersey but spent most of her life in North Carolina with her sister, Kristen, and parents. She earned a B.S. in chemistry from Western Carolina University in 2003, and her M.Ed. in Secondary Education from Jones International University in 2010. She has a wonderful relationship with her fur-babies and saltwater fish. In her spare time, Heather enjoys the outdoors and Steeler football!

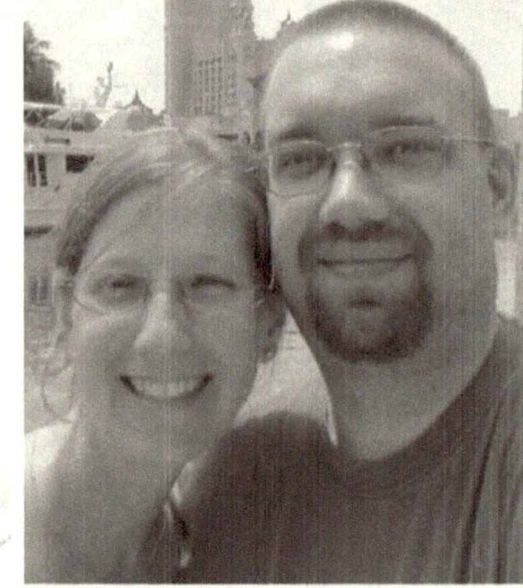

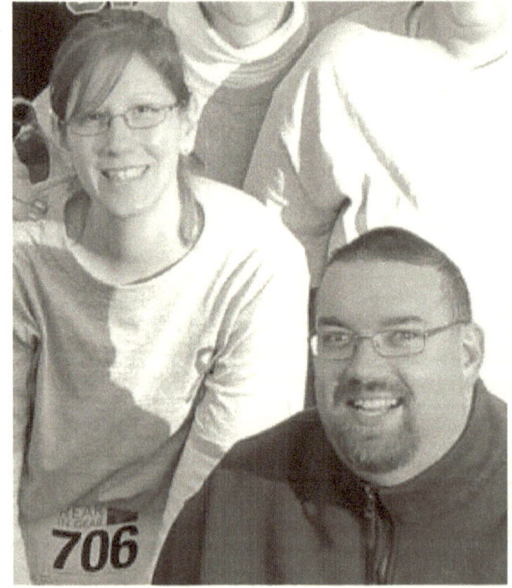

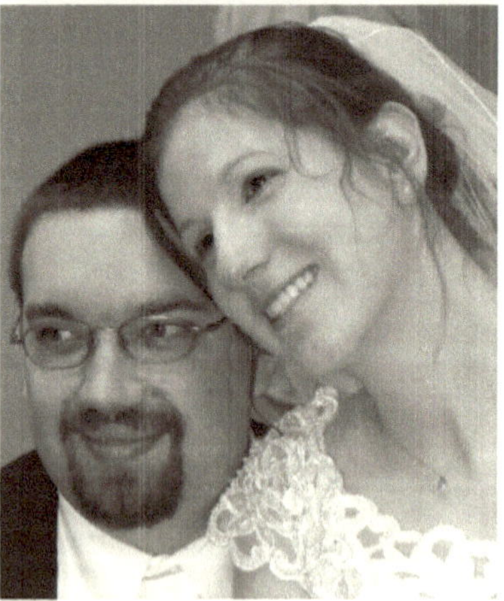

*

SUE NOVA
Sue's husband Dana died from
lung cancer in 2012 at age 46

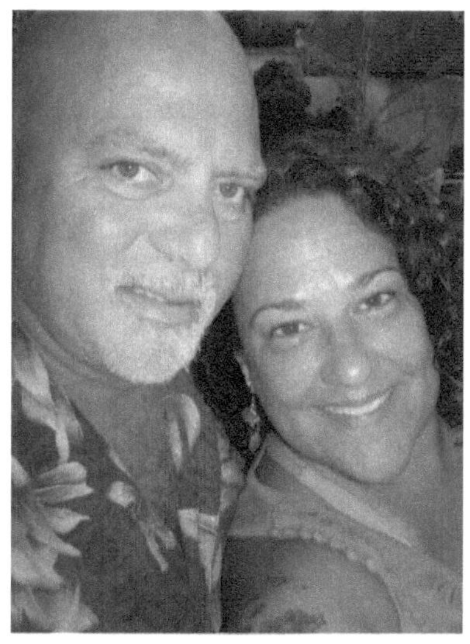

Sue Nova found the love of her life and had planned to grow old with this man. Her life, as she knew it, ended the day that man took his last breath. At forty-nine years old she had to learn how to live without him. She had to learn to move through the grief that enveloped her. She had to learn how to live without her heart. At fifty-three years old she picked up and left everything she knew and moved to a different state. That was where she decided to start a new life. There was no judgment there. No one knew her story. No one knew her past. It was in her new place, with a new tribe that she was finally able to shed the old and begin to live.

*

SHERYL POCHEL
Sheryl's husband Brian died from
pancreatic cancer in 2011 at age 43

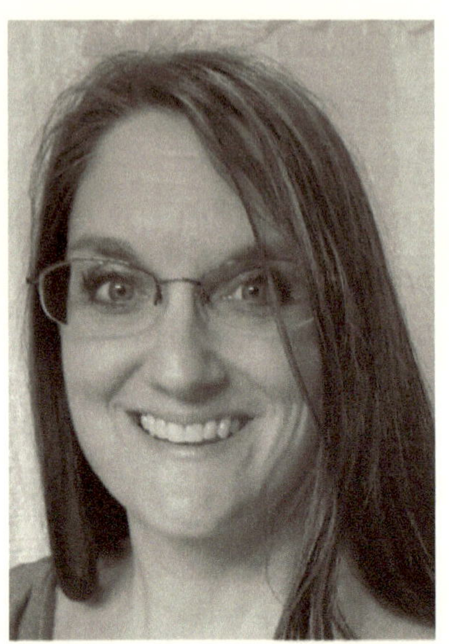

Shortly after her husband's cancer diagnosis, in which they were given little to no hope for his survival, her best friend said to one of her friends "Sheryl is the happiest person I know. Her husband is dying, and she is still the happiest person I have ever met." While that statement may not always be true, for the most part it is pretty descriptive.

Sheryl is an only parent of four kids, ages thirteen to eighteen, living in the village of Cottage Grove, Wisconsin, where she and her husband owned his chiropractic practice. After her husband's death from pancreatic cancer, it took her a while to figure out what she wanted to do for a living, since she worked for him at his clinic. Having an M.S. degree in Home Economics with an emphasis in apparel design, she decided to use her design skills and became a home stager. She is currently self employed as a certified home stager and owns Inside Story Staging, LLC

*

KATHIE SCOTT
Kathie's 57-year-old husband Jim
died from prostate cancer in 2009

Kathie recently retired from her local police department as their Communications Supervisor and is in the process of finding her way in the retirement world. She is the mother of three grown daughters and four grandchildren. Kathie has been a working mother all of her adult life so this adventure into retirement is an interesting one for sure!

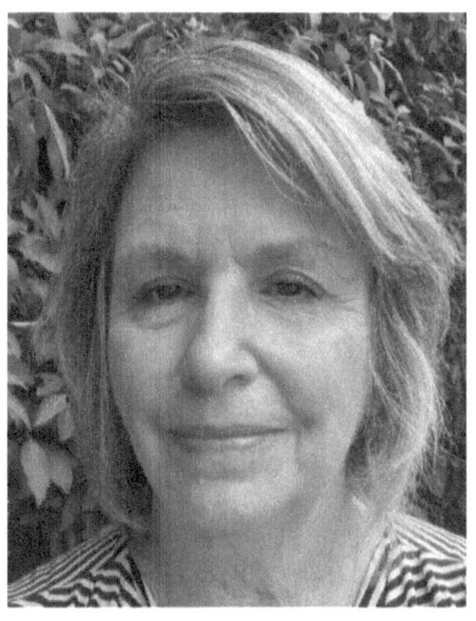

*
STEVE SHARP
Steve's 51-year-old wife Carolyn
died from melanoma in 2014

Steve Sharp was born in Lewisburg, Pennsylvania, and grew up in Virginia Beach. He earned his B.S. in Computer Science from Old Dominion University and his M.S. in Systems Engineering from George Mason University. Steve was married in 1980 to Jean Treynor, with whom he had three children, Beth, Matthew and David. Jean worked as a registered nurse until she became ill with a chronic disease in 1989, contributing to her death from congestive heart failure in January 1999. Steve met Carolyn Smith, a widow, online in December 1999, and then met in person at a group for young widows and widower in Virginia Beach. He married her in July 2000. Carolyn brought two children into the marriage, Kenny and Holly. Carolyn was a high

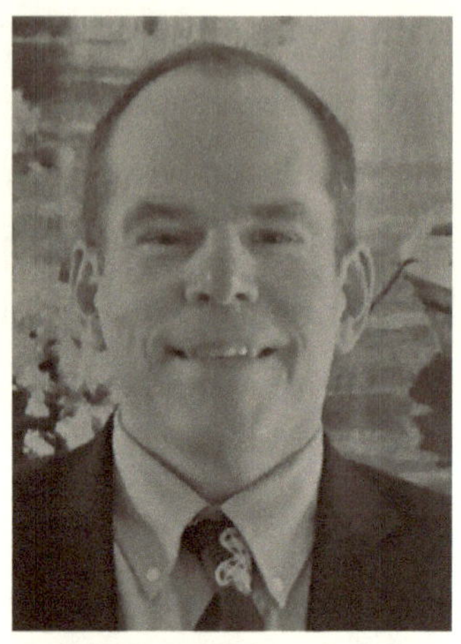

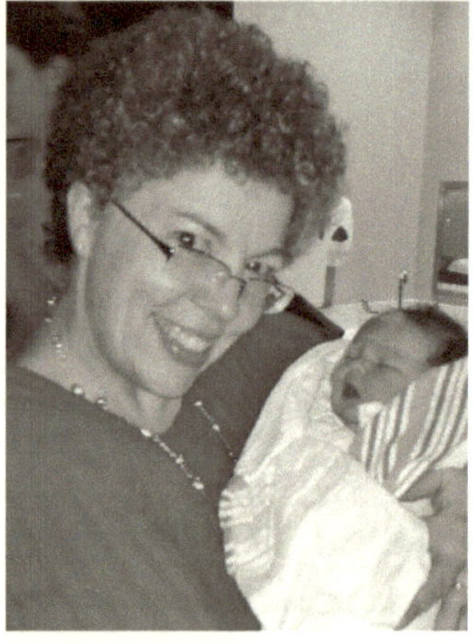

school chemistry teacher and touched many young people with her compassion for learning and her concern for their welfare. Carolyn was diagnosed with stage IV melanoma in August 2013, and passed away in October 2014. Steve married Julia Wallace in May 2017. Between them they have seven children and seven grandchildren. Steve enjoys playing French horn for his church, biking, and traveling to new destinations.

*

STEPHANIE VANDERVALK
Stephanie's husband Rob died from
osteosarcoma in 2016 at age 24

Stephanie was born in London, Ontario, the youngest of three siblings. At age two, her family moved to Cambridge, Ontario where she currently resides. Stephanie has always had a desire for helping others, which directed her to study Registered Nursing at McMaster University. She has an enormous passion for those in palliative care, where she wishes to pursue her career as a registered nurse.

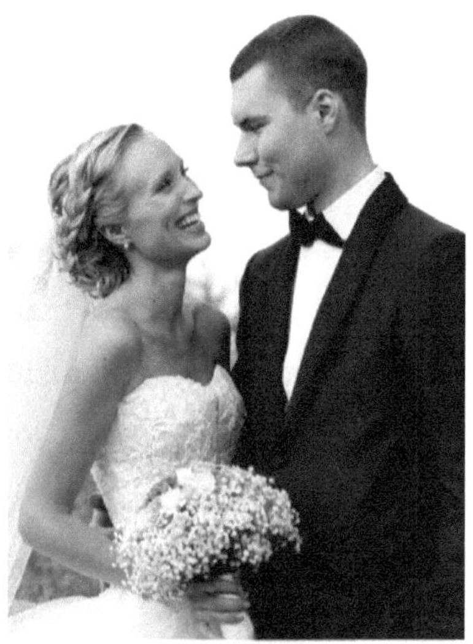

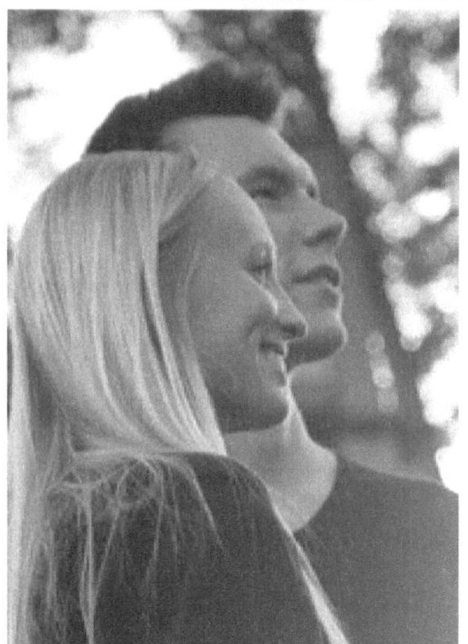

*
DIANNE WEST
Dianne's husband Vern died from
multiple myeloma in 2010 at age 69

Originally from a small town in southeast
Michigan, Dianne married at eighteen and
was blessed to share forty-one years with
her husband, Vern. She was his caregiver
for over four years as he fought multiple
myeloma, a blood cancer that attacks the
bone marrow. Widowed in 2010, Dianne
has dedicated her post-loss life to
volunteering within the widowed
community. She is the National Volunteer
Coordinator for Soaring Spirits
International, a nonprofit organization
committed to providing resources and peer
support to people who have lost a spouse
or life partner. Dianne is the Widowed
Village administrator, a member of the
Camp Widow Leadership Team, oversees

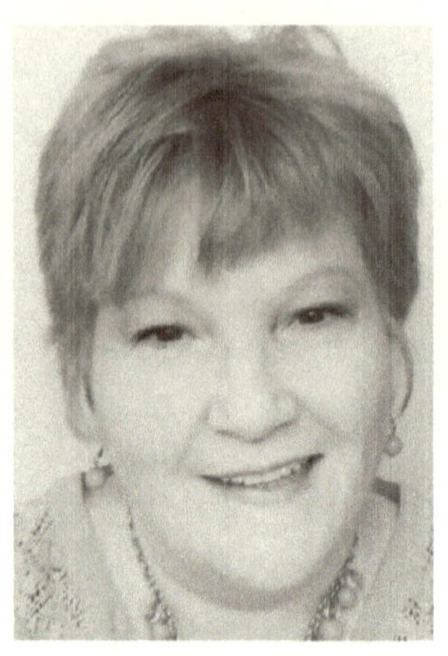

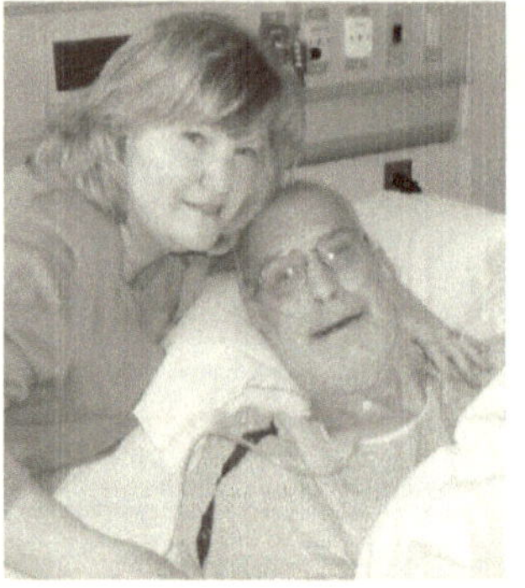

the Soaring Spirits Regional Group program, and leads a regional
group in the Las Vegas area. She retired from the Las Vegas Valley
Water District in 2015 after twenty-nine years of service, and is the
owner of Tending Your Heart and Soul where she teaches the Brave
Girls Soul Restoration curriculum as a certified instructor. Dianne
coauthored Grief Diaries: Surviving the Loss of a Spouse and
contributed to Grief Diaries: How to Help the Newly Bereaved.

FROM LYNDA CHELDELIN FELL

Thank you

I am deeply indebted to the writers who contributed to this book. It required tremendous courage to pen such painful memories for the purpose of helping others, and the collective effort is a legacy to be proud of. I'm humbled to partner with coauthor Dianne West, a lovely lady who is dedicated to plowing the field and planting seeds of hope for grievers everywhere.

I greatly appreciate our Grief Diaries village and the lovely souls I consider dear friends, collaborative partners, mentors, and muses. I treasure each and every one of you! Finally, it goes without saying how thankful I am for my husband Jamie, our children, and our wonderful family and friends for being there through laughter and tears.

Helen Keller once said, "Walking with a friend in the dark is better than walking alone in the light." By sharing our struggles, we learn that we aren't truly alone as we travel our journey, for there are others ahead of us, behind us, and right beside us. That is what Grief Diaries is all about.

Lynda Cheldelin Fell

Shared joy is doubled joy;
shared sorrow is half a sorrow.
SWEDISH PROVERB

*

ABOUT

LYNDA CHELDELIN FELL

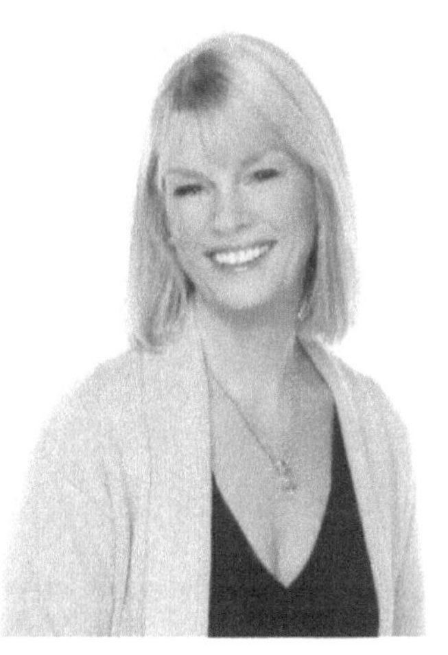

Considered a pioneer in the field of inspirational hope in the aftermath of loss, Lynda Cheldelin Fell has a passion for producing groundbreaking projects that create a legacy of help, healing, and hope.

She is co-founder of the International Grief Institute, CEO of AlyBlue Media, and creator of the award-winning Grief Diaries and Real Life Diaries book series. Her repertoire of interviews include Dr. Martin Luther King's daughter, Trayvon Martin's mother, sisters of the late Nicole Brown Simpson, Pastor Todd Burpo of Heaven Is For Real, and other societal newsmakers on finding healing and hope in the aftermath of life's harshest challenges. She has earned four national literary awards and is a current nominee for five national 2017 advocacy awards.

Lynda's own story began in 2007, when she had an alarming dream about her young teenage daughter, Aly. In the dream, Aly was a backseat passenger in a car that veered off the road and sailed into a lake. Aly sank with the car, leaving behind an open book floating face down on the water. Two years later, Lynda's dream became reality when her daughter was killed as a backseat passenger in a car accident while coming home from a swim meet. Overcome with grief, Lynda's forty-six-year-old husband suffered a major stroke that left him with severe disabilities, changing the family dynamics once again.

The following year, Lynda was invited to share her remarkable story about finding hope after loss, and she accepted. That cathartic experience inspired her to create groundbreaking projects spanning national events, radio, film and books to help others who share the same journey feel less alone. Now considered one of the foremost grief educators and healing facilitators in the United States, Lynda is dedicated to helping ordinary people share their own stories of survival and hope in the aftermath of loss.

lynda@lyndafell.com | www.lyndafell.com

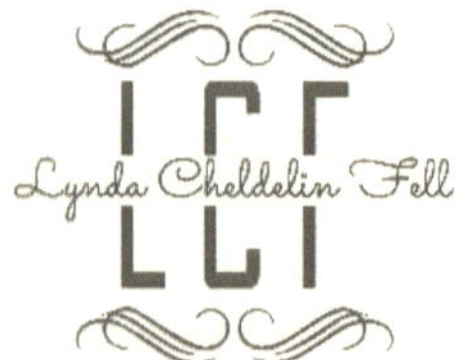

ALYBLUE MEDIA TITLES

Grief Diaries: Victim Impact Statement

Grief Diaries: Hit by Impaired Driver

Grief Diaries: Surviving Loss of a Spouse

Grief Diaries: Surviving Loss of a Child

Grief Diaries: Surviving Loss of a Sibling

Grief Diaries: Surviving Loss of a Parent

Grief Diaries: Surviving Loss of an Infant

Grief Diaries: Surviving Loss of a Loved One

Grief Diaries: Surviving Loss by Suicide

Grief Diaries: Surviving Loss of Health

Grief Diaries: How to Help the Newly Bereaved

Grief Diaries: Loss by Impaired Driving

Grief Diaries: Loss by Homicide

Grief Diaries: Loss of a Pregnancy

Grief Diaries: Hello from Heaven

Grief Diaries: Grieving for the Living

Grief Diaries: Shattered

Grief Diaries: Project Cold Case

Grief Diaries: Poetry & Prose and More

Grief Diaries: Through the Eyes of Men

Grief Diaries: Will We Survive?

Real Life Diaries: Living with a Brain Injury

Real Life Diaries: Through the Eyes of DID

Real Life Diaries: Through the Eyes of an Eating Disorder

Real Life Diaries: Living with Endometriosis

Real Life Diaries: Living with Mental Illness

Real Life Diaries: Through the Eyes of a Funeral Director

Grammy Visits From Heaven

Grandpa Visits From Heaven

Faith, Grief & Pass the Chocolate Pudding

Heaven Talks to Children

Color My Soul Whole

A Child is Missing: A True Story

A Child is Missing: Searching for Justice

Grief Reiki

Humanity's legacy of stories and storytelling
is the most precious we have.

DORIS LESSING

*

To share your story, visit
www.griefdiaries.com
www.RealLifeDiaries.com

PUBLISHED BY ALYBLUE MEDIA
Inside every human is a story worth sharing.
www.AlyBlueMedia.com

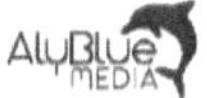

SURVIVING LOSS BY CANCER